CU00951247

Crossroads to Cure

The Homoeopath's Guide

to

Second Prescription

NICOLA HENRIQUES

TOTALITY PRESS

Published by Totality Press
1336-D Oak Avenue
St. Helena, CA 94574

© Totality Press 1998

All rights reserved. No part of this book may be reproduced
in any form or by any means, electronic or mechanical,
including photocopy, recording, or any information storage
or retrieval system, without permission in writing
from the publisher.

Printed in the United States of America

02 01   5 4 3 2

Cover design by Nola Burger
Cover artwork by Stephen Henriques

Library of Congress Catalog Card Number

98-61078

Publishers Cataloging-in-Publication
(*Provided by Quality Books, Inc.*)

Henriques, Nicola.

Crossroads to cure : the homoeopath's guide to second
prescription / Nicola Henriques—1st ed.

p. cm.

Includes bibliographical references and index.
Preassigned LCCN 98-
ISBN 0-9663388-0-4

1. Homoeopathy—Materia medica and therapeutics   1. Title.

RX621.H46 1998   615.5'32
                                  QBI98-924

CROSSROADS TO CURE

TO ALL THOSE WHO LABOR TO RELIEVE
THE SUFFERING OF OTHERS

CONTENTS

About The Author

Nicola Henriques is a British homoeopath and author of six books, now living and teaching in the United States. She graduated from the London College of Classical Homoeopathy, had a busy London practice, and ran a free clinic within the National Health Service, before moving to California to become principal lecturer at the Institute of Classical Homoeopathy, San Francisco. Her other books include *Menopause, The Woman's View* and *Hysterectomy, The Woman's View,* both published by Quartet Books, London.

Crossroads to Cure is the first of three books by Ms. Henriques to be published by Totality Press.

ACKNOWLEDGEMENTS

I WISH TO THANK THE FOLLOWING friends and colleagues for their important and very individual contributions to the publication of this book. Cara Landry, Institute of Classical Homoeopathy (ICH), Program Director, for inviting me to come and teach in California; her inspiration for this, the first in a series of ICH guidebooks to classical homoeopathy, and her editorial support. Anne Dickson, long time friend, for introducing me to homoeopath Misha Norland, whose explanation of what homoeopaths do resulted in my quitting journalism and training to become a professional, classical homoeopath. Sheilagh Creasy, scholar and practitioner of homoeopathy, whose teaching led me through the maze of homoeopathic literature to what she called the "good books" of the great Hahnemannian homoeopaths. Rosemary Wood, who did the difficult work of organizing material and quote checking. Susanna Dakin, for her critical eye and detailed suggestions. Sharon Chelton, for skillfully and quickly typing the first draft manuscript. Stephanie Bero, for her invaluable "lay person" critiques and manuscript production. Linda Baer of Padma Publishing for typesetting the book. Anna Smith of Padma Publishing for proofreading. Stephen Henriques, artist and recently discovered jazz cousin, for so kindly contributing the beautiful, original artwork for the jacket design created by Nola Burger. Greatest thanks to my main man, Sam. Finally, I express my grateful appreciation to all the ICH students, whose challenging, insatiable thirst for clarity on this complex, vital topic, as well as their thought-provoking questions, inspired me to labor with love and find answers.

Author's Preface

PRIOR TO TAKING UP THE STUDY of homoeopathy, I was for many years a writer and journalistic researcher. It was while researching for two books about hysterectomy and menopause that I began to seriously question my view of health and disease.

My investigations into the dominant medical management of the mental and physical turmoil of menopause brought me to the dead end of hysterectomy and/or hormone replacement therapy. I thought that surgery, removing probably the most intimate and integral part of a woman's body, or long-term drug therapy couldn't be the only roads to health. For some reason I believed there had to be gentler, more creative, and dare I say it, more compassionate routes worthy of consideration and application during this natural transition.

This strong desire to discover alternative routes led me directly to the field of Complementary Medicine. Significantly the word "complementary" means to complete, *to make whole,* an extremely appropriate concept to bring to mind when discussing holistic, vitalistic systems of medicine such as acupuncture, osteopathy, chiropractic, traditional Chinese medicine, massage, and of course homoeopathy.

Contrary to dominant medical practice that treats a single troubled part in isolation from the rest of the person, *complementary* holistic systems of medicine restore balance, health, and optimum function, by perceiving and treating the human organism as a whole, complete unit, comprising physical, mental, and emotional levels, vitality, and spirit. Having discovered the "complementary" view of health, disease, and cure, to ascertain the efficacy of the different medical models in the treatment of menopause, I set about interviewing several leading practitioners in different fields, among them Misha Norland, the well-known British homoeopath. After he explained how homoeopathic medicine effectively and rapidly readjusts the internal imbalance manifest in menopausal symptoms, I asked him what exactly he did in order to find the right medicine for each separate individual.

The answer triggered a wave of excitement such as I had never, ever experienced before. Like Saul on the road to Damascus, suddenly everything changed and I saw what I should be doing with the rest of my life! Misha kindly contributed to the menopause book, and as soon as I could, I stopped full-time writing and began full-time study of homoeopathy.

A deeply skeptical, down to earth, practical person by nature, through study I sought to penetrate the mist of myth, magic, and mystery that prevails about homoeopathy. This book is an attempt to break through existing misunderstandings, and comes from my experience as homoeopathic student, patient, practitioner, and later teacher in Britain and America.

The project started during my training, when along with some of my student colleagues, I was extremely frustrated by inconsistent confusing responses to questions about what exactly happens when a homoeopathic medicine is administered and why. What is it exactly practitioners look for during the first and subsequent progress report interviews? How exactly do patients and practitioners know if and how well the remedy acted, and how do they decide what to do next?

To come to the deepest understanding of homoeopathy and how it works, I needed to carefully scrutinize the critically important so-called "second prescription" phase of the homoeopathic healing process. After all, it is at this point we decide the patient is getting worse, better, or staying the same. So what is the concrete evidence upon which we base such decisions and how is it best obtained?

In Britain when attending the school clinic and while observing different homoeopaths, I saw a wide variety of patient evaluation procedures in action. Although interesting and intriguing, most of them failed in terms of clarity, guidance, and consistency regarding *what* I could expect to happen with treatment: *how* to analyze the remedy action, *why* certain changes occurred, and *how* to proceed with treatment. The kind of person who enjoys getting to the bottom of things, in my heart I knew that hidden somewhere within the sometimes difficult language of the original and early homoeopathic texts there must be a clearly defined logic for assessing and analyzing the progress of each case.

Utilizing my professional research skills, I sought out solid, proven second prescription information from those closest to the original source of homoeopathy, Hahnemann and his early followers who repeatedly proved the efficacy of his simple systematic method of homoeopathic practice. Studying the literary legacy of the consistently classical "master" homoeopaths from the olden days gradually cleared the mist. I was relieved to discover that everything I needed to know about the complex task of ongoing case management, including making the crucial second prescription, had been carefully documented here and there in many different works. In this book I have unearthed and gathered together their information for a coherent patient progress evaluation method, which helps prevent many common case management mistakes and leads to astonishingly effective treatment.

I hope the information presented in these pages relieves frustrations, demystifies, and brings about a clear understanding of the natural and powerful self-curative process of the awe-inspiring life force. I hope the book benefits patients and practitioners equally and hastens both toward the rapid restoration of health.

Nicola Henriques
Institute of Classical Homoeopathy
San Francisco, USA
June, 1998

INTRODUCTION

WHETHER AMATEUR PRESCRIBER, beginning practitioner, or well-known professional homoeopath, who amongst us hasn't at some time struggled to answer the questions: Has the remedy acted and is it still acting? How long should I watch and wait? Is the patient experiencing new symptoms, a return of original (presenting) symptoms, or old symptoms from the past? Is there such a thing as the "standstill" phase? Why hasn't the patient responded to a well-indicated remedy?

When was the last time you racked your brain struggling for clarity in a situation where patient and symptoms suddenly went haywire, or the patient suddenly went into a serious, rapid decline and you didn't know why or what to do next? All these questions and ponderings amount to what is probably the most difficult aspect of homoeopathic treatment, when and how to make the successful *second prescription*.

Drawing on the most reliable classical sources, this book endeavors to lead the reader step by step through the complicated process of evaluation and decision-making after the first homoeopathic prescription has been made. In this book you will find the most common remedy action scenarios accompanied by evaluation criteria and recommendations for further action and the philosophical principles on which they are based. I have quoted liberally from the classical sources and, for the sake of fluency, have also paraphrased quotes within the text, giving the references so that the reader may seek out the exact wording.

If you are a practitioner or student, this book will serve as a guide and constant companion. If you use homoeopathy, caring for your family's first aid needs, or are a homoeopathic patient seeking to understand your therapeutic process, this book will give you practical guidance and a clear understanding of homoeopathy.

At the moment of the second prescription, patients are at a critical crossroad in treatment. Since everything rests upon the practitioner's understanding of exactly what has happened to the patient after administration of the first prescription, success or failure to cure is in delicate balance. For some, the second prescription is the phase of homoeopathic practice that causes the greatest anxiety, consternation, and confusion. To avoid its becoming the biggest obstacle to cure calls for artistry and skill.

When decisions are made following the fundamental principles of *classical* homoeopathic practice, the second prescription treatment phase is the moment that holds the greatest promise of truly healing the sick, as Hahnemann instructs, gently, rapidly, and permanently. In modern practice we are faced with increasingly complicated cases, the result of lifelong suppressive treatment* and the inevitable imbalances of stressful lifestyles.

---

* See pages 27–28 for explanation of suppression.

To reduce suffering, homoeopathic practitioners must possess the most comprehensive understanding of our healing art. In this regard, to be successful, it is extremely important to be conscious of what we rely on to guide our understanding and decisions during the second prescription evaluation process. Should we rely solely on intuition, the vagaries of our psychic abilities, and forget logical thinking?

> If you talk with a great many physicians concerning the observations you have made after giving the remedy you will find that the majority of them have only whims or notions on this subject and see nothing after the prescription is made.[1]

Surely, for the patient's sake, we should better rely on something with substance; something with a proven track record of success utilized by great homoeopaths again and again in every imaginable circumstance—Hahnemann's clearly comprehensible, fundamental principles of practice. Far from being someone's pet theory, they originate and have their roots in ancient medical and philosophical writings. Their application was researched and developed by the founder and the greatest practitioner/teacher of homoeopathy, Dr. Samuel Hahnemann. They are explained in his *Organon of Medicine* and were practiced with confidence and tremendous success by his dedicated students and followers including Boenninghausen, Hering, Kent, Dunham, Close, the Farringtons, Wright-Hubbard, and many others.

Confronted daily with perplexing situations, wouldn't it be wonderful to be able to phone, fax, e-mail, and download any of these great practitioners for quick, calm advice on how to unravel confusion and rapidly reduce the patient's suffering?

In the present climate of impatience and constant rush to develop "new improved" versions of everything, let's not risk ignoring the meticulous, valuable work of the great, past masters of classical homoeopathy. Jam-packed with precious jewels of information, their wealth of writings are based on a clever combination of the clearest understanding of Hahnemann's work, together with their own massive clinical experience and careful research.* True scientists don't reject past experience; they build on what has gone before and try to come to a greater understanding of it. No one need revolutionize or reinvent the homoeopathic wheel. The comprehensive work of these great practitioner/ teachers is as valuable today as it was when written and forms the firmest foundation on which to build the classical homoeopathy of the future. As Kent eloquently put it:

> Some of experience make lesser blunders and some make few, but how many have made none? All these blunders I have made, as I had

---

* As an example, see the low versus high potency prescription experiment conducted at Leopoldstadt Hospital, Vienna from 1850 to 1859, described in Dunham's *Homoeopathy, the Science of Therapeutics*.

no teacher, until I blundered upon the works of the great Master.[2]

Practicing homoeopathy without the guidance of our most experienced and successful predecessors, we are travelers without a map, wandering aimlessly about, unable to reach our destination. Such confusion is a disaster for the patient. If we carefully examine Hahnemann's expert system we'll find all the clarity and tools necessary for the restoration of health to people the world over and once again raise confidence in the efficacy of homoeopathy.

In the current worldwide resurgence of interest in homoeopathy, it is vital to remember that homoeopathy itself is constantly being judged. In all aspects of practice, as homoeopaths of today and tomorrow we hold in our hands the success or failure of Dr. Samuel Hahnemann's simple, scientific, complete, and beneficial system of medicine. As he says in the *Organon*:

> Thus homoeopathy is a perfectly simple system of medicine, remaining always fixed in its principles as in its practice, which, like the doctrine whereon it is based, if rightly apprehended will be found to be complete and therefore serviceable.[3]*

To let the voices of the great masters ring in your ears and to help you make accurate and effective second prescriptions, I humbly offer this work and passionately

---

* Preface to the *Organon*. Most quotes are from the sixth edition of this work, translated by Boericke.

urge you to take up the precision tools of your trade: The *original* works of Hahnemann and his early followers. Study for the first time or reacquaint yourself with their writings. Let them become to you, as they have become to me, reliable, true friends and colleagues. I guarantee, in your hour of need, they'll never let you down.

INTRODUCTION

1. Kent, *Lectures on Homoeopathic Philosophy*, Lecture 35, pg. 244.
2. Kent, *Minor Writings,* pg. 236.
3. Hahnemann, *Organon,* 6th ed. (Boericke trans.), Preface, pg. 19.

CHAPTER 1

Golden Keys

WHETHER THE PRACTITIONER is embarking on taking the case and making the first prescription or struggling with second prescription questions and difficulties, the greatest asset is to understand fully how it is that homoeopathy actually works. Far from being some random mystical thing, homoeopathy is a beautifully logical, practical, and proven science. Hahnemann has given us the golden keys to understanding homoeopathic practice in a set of principles.

In the first sentence of his brilliant lectures on homoeopathic philosophy, Kent states that there are principles that govern the practice of homoeopathic medicine. He goes on to say:

> Hahnemann has given us principles that we can study and advance upon. It is law that governs the world and not matters of opinion or hypothesis. We must begin by having a respect for law, for we have no starting point unless we base our propositions on law.[1]

Understanding the fundamental principles of homoeopathy is the essence of effective homoeopathic medicine. They are applied in taking the case accurately, when selecting remedies and optimum potency, and they play a crucial role in the second prescription treatment phase, especially the management of complex cases. Successful cure depends on understanding that disease is a change of state by degree from harmony to disharmony, requiring logical thinking and application of *all* the principles. Careful reading of Hahnemann's *Organon of Medicine* reveals that these principles are the underlying structure of the homoeopathic system of medicine, governing all its aspects. They are explained further in Hahnemann's *Chronic Diseases* and in the works of Hering, Kent, Roberts, Close, and Dunham.

In brief, the principles underpinning classical homoeopathic practice are as follows:

Vital Force (Also Called the Life Principle)

> In the healthy condition of man, the spiritual vital force . . . the dynamis that animates the material body (organism), rules with unbounded sway, and retains all parts of the organism in admirable, harmonious vital operation . . .[2]

The vital force gives life to any organism. Known as *chi* in Chinese medicine, the Life Force is the energy system of the body responsible for maintaining the harmonious healthy function of the organism.* When life is threatened to any degree, in its effort to maintain bal-

---

* See definition of "life," *Webster's International Dictionary*, Merriam and Company, London and Massachusetts, 1902: "The potential principle or force by which the organs of animals and plants are started and continued in the

ance and harmonious function, the vital force attempts to banish disorder from the interior to the exterior boundaries of the body. This life preserving activity inevitably produces uncomfortable sensations, which we call symptoms.

In homoeopathy, symptoms are considered curative because they are not only the means by which the vital force attempts to throw off the energetic pattern of disharmony we know as disease, but also they act as a vent and soothe the distressed vital force. Symptoms are also the language of the disordered vital force. They signal the precise nature and character of the individual's distress, thereby indicating through the Law of Similars and reference to the materia medica, the remedy required for that particular individual at that particular time, in that particular change of state.

In the second prescription phase, evaluating the action of the previous remedy and the state of the vital force, as manifest through symptoms is our only guide to the next action. Lose sight of the signs of the vital force, ignore or misinterpret them, and we are lost and cannot help the patient.

Susceptibility

The patient's susceptibility is the second principle to play an essential role in health, disease, and cure from a homoeopathic perspective. The best way to un-

performance of their several and cooperative functions."
Also see Paragraphs 9 through 13, Hahnemann's *Organon of Medicine,* sixth edition.

derstand the principle of susceptibility is first, look at the definition of the word itself.

The dictionary defines susceptibility as: a state or quality of being susceptible to stimuli; the capability of receiving impressions; the power to react.

The key words here are: *state, quality, receiving, reacting.* Not mentioned is the word *degree,* another very important word to use because, according to our susceptibility, everything is experienced in *degree* at any one moment. For example, susceptibility is the degree to which the human organism is affected internally and externally by something and to what degree the effect is positive or negative. Trauma, environment, changes in temperature, diet, how we react to offense, loss, love, joy, all manner of life circumstances are examples of stimuli to which we are variously susceptible. According to the Law of Similars, in homoeopathy cure takes place because we are as similarly susceptible to the homoeopathic medicine as we are to the stimulus that disturbed us.

The way we may know or perceive the existence of such a thing as susceptibility is through the way the individual responds, reacts, and adapts to various internal and external stimuli. In other words, susceptibility is about how well we adapt to and survive in a variety of situations and stresses to which we are constantly exposed throughout life. Among other things, it enables us to breathe and digest food, experience loving relationships, and roll with the punches. So, as we can see, susceptibility is the basis of balanced life and health.

In the homoeopathic context, susceptibility is the degree of the reactivity of the life force and is a quality or state of the vital force at a given moment. It could be said, if the vital force is a face, susceptibility is the expression on the face, they are so integrated.

The true state of balance or disturbance of the patient's life force and susceptibility is perceived in the case taking, as the patient tells his story of disease through the experience of symptoms. In the context of his life circumstances and symptom patterns, we perceive each individual's state of vital force and susceptibility and the ability or inability to adapt appropriately to all kinds of stimuli. Perceiving the vital force in its state of susceptibility enables homoeopaths to determine the strength of the individual's defense mechanism and the strength of the disturbance.

Miasms

In homoeopathy, according to Hahnemann, the underlying causation of pathology or suffering is due to each individual's predominating miasms. Miasm, from the Greek word for defilement or pollution, is the characteristic inherited tendency to be susceptible to certain diseases.

Carrying on the ideas of ancient physicians and philosophers regarding the nature of individual constitutions, to the homoeopath Hahnemann's concept of miasms answers the nagging questions, when did the disease begin, what is its source, and why do patients fall ill over and over again? After fifteen years of extensive research and analysis, Hahnemann came to the understanding that disease was caused by some inherent, unceasing, latent influence residing in the organism. Occasionally in balance, we free ourselves from this influence—"I'm healthy again" we cry, but eventually it returns as if in a new garment or disguise, always somewhat changed in its expression of action or character. The business of these miasms is to constantly attempt to tear down and murder life through multiple underproductive, overproductive, and destructive processes, which combine to make gaps and breaches in nature that a debilitated life force cannot repair. As Allen writes in his book, *The Chronic Miasms and Pseudo-Psora,* Hahnemann believed miasms to be related to and stem from the major disease patterns affecting the human race throughout its history, which have left their indelible mark on our inheritance. The activity of these inherited, ultimately destructive disease traits are indicated by the individual's pattern of disease, as portrayed by the expression of symptoms and family medical history.

There are four defined miasms: *psoric,* which is the inhibitory, underproductive tendency; *syphilitic,* the destructive tendency; and *sycotic,* the excessive, overproductive tendency. The fourth, *tubercular* tendency, derives from a marriage of underproduction and destruction tendencies resulting in a wasting self-consuming tendency. From a homoeopathic perspective, disorders resulting in cancer and AIDS derive from a complex, compounding of all four major miasms.

In homoeopathy, the vital force, susceptibility, and miasms are an intangible, inseparable dynamic trio that comprises the living organism. In order to select the correct remedy for a specific change of state in an individual, including alternations of states, classical homoeopaths apply the miasm principle when viewing an individual's disease symptom image or pattern, because certain remedy actions express aspects of one or several miasmatic tendencies.

The Law of Similars

> That which has the power to harm, has the power to heal. (*Hippocrates*)

In their uniquely prepared, dynamized state, homoeopathic medicines act as similar, dynamic, *artificial* forms of disease *simulating* the patient's *original* (natural) disease. Hahnemann explained their mode of action in Paragraphs 26, 27, and 34 of the *Organon:*

> In the living organism a weaker dynamic affection is permanently extinguished by a stronger one if the latter (deviating in kind) is very similar in its manifestations to the former . . . Therefore, the healing power of medicines rests upon their faculty of producing symptoms similar to the disease, and superior to it in strength, so that each individual case of disease is most certainly, fundamentally, and rapidly extinguished and cancelled by a drug which is more potent than the disease, and capable of producing in the body symptoms most similar to, and completely resembling the totality of those of the disease.[3]

Dynamization of homoeopathic medicines renders them energetically stronger than the original disease. Dynamization also allows the energetic properties of the medicine to act directly on the susceptibility of the energetic vital force. They target and resemble the state of the vital force, correspond to the predominant miasm, and satisfy the patient's susceptibility. The helping hand of homoeopathic remedies enables the vital force to overcome the original natural disease and restore equilibrium.

Provings

A true scientist, Hahnemann realized that to know the curative potential and power of medicines they needed to be tested. Provings are conducted according to strict protocols established by Hahnemann and laid out in the *Organon*. Hahnemann's medicinal provings were the first systematically conducted drug tests and the precursor to today's mainstream medicine drug trials. To demonstrate and prove the range of medicinal effectiveness he carried out extensive, carefully documented provings on himself, his family, and colleagues. Repeated doses of a remedy were given to *healthy* people and relevant data was scientifically collected by documenting what symptoms were produced. In this way he discovered what symptoms each medicine has the power to induce and, through the Law of Similars, what symptom totality in the sick person the medicine is capable of curing. Proving data is collected in the homoeopathic materia medica.

> [Homoeopathy] employs for cure *only* those medicines whose power for altering and deranging (dynamically) the health it knows *accurately,* and from these it selects one whose pathogenetic power (its medicinal disease) is

capable of removing the natural disease in question by similarity (*similia similibus*) . . .[4]

In second prescription deliberations, reference to and utilization of data collected from the provings plays a significant role in evaluating the old, presenting, or new symptoms that occur and how they relate to the curative potential of the selected remedy.

Succussion and Dilution

Since in homoeopathy we always seek to perceive and select the optimum dosage of medicine needed to act on the dynamic vital force and restore balance, it is necessary to thoroughly understand the principle of Succussion and Dilution. This is the potentiation preparation method of homoeopathic medicines. Ultimately, accurate selection of dosage and potency play an essential role in the homoeopathic healing process.

The simplest way to explain this principle is to substitute the word *dynamization* for Succussion and *attenuation* for Dilution, and then look at the dictionary definition of these words. According to Webster's 1902 edition, *dynamization* is the act of setting free the dynamic powers of a medicine as by shaking the bottle containing it. Succussion, therefore, means agitating, shaking, or striking the medicine container, resulting in the dynamization of homoeopathic medicines.

Attenuation is the process by mechanical or chemical action of breaking inanimate substances down into finer parts, making them less dense, (diluting them), making them less complex. Through serial dilution and succussion inanimate substances are rendered easily ac-

cessible to the ultimate target of homoeopathic medicine, the dynamic vital force. The Law of Similars is applied again because in homoeopathy, disease and homoeopathic remedies are both dynamic.

In the second prescription evaluation process, accuracy of preceding remedy dosage is considered when assessing whether or not a remedy has worked and has
exhausted its action, or whether it has overacted in a
highly susceptible individual, or whether a remedy has
not acted because the dosage did not accurately match
the state of the dynamic trio in the first place.

Minimum Dose

As in choosing the first prescription, selection of
the second prescription demands adherence to Hahnemann's instruction to administer the *single remedy* in
the *minimum dose* required to effect the curative response.

In no case under treatment is it necessary and
therefore not permissible to administer to a patient more than *one single, simple medicinal*
substance at one time. It is inconceivable how
the slightest doubt could exist as to whether it
was more consistent with nature and more ra-
tional to prescribe a *single, simple* medicine at
one time in a disease or a mixture of several
differently acting drugs. It is absolutely not allowed in homoeopathy, the one true, simple
and natural art of healing, to give the patient *at
one time* two different medicinal substances.[5]

He instructs *minimum potency* to effect cure thus:

> [Homoeopathy] administers to the patient in
> simple form, but in rare and minute doses so
> small that, without occasioning pain or weak-
> ening, they just suffice to remove the natural
> malady . . .[6]

Classical homoeopaths give a single remedy and
never mix or compound medicines for several other logical reasons: the experimental work in constructing the
homoeopathic materia medica has been conducted with
single medicines, and as each medicine has its own definite and peculiar kind and sphere of action, scientific
accuracy, as well as the Law of Similars, requires that
the treatment be conducted in the same manner.

Furthermore, as Hahnemann states in the *Organon,* Paragraph 274, even though the single medicines
were thoroughly proved on the healthy, it is impossible
to predict how two and more medicinal substances,
when compounded, might hinder and alter each other's
actions. Also, the action of homoeopathic remedies
given singly is complete and unchanged by the action of
other medicines.

The final reason for giving a single remedy lies in
the fact that our prescriptions are based on knowledge
of both the individual's symptom image totality and the
proven symptom image of the single remedy, leading to
selection of a single remedy for a single individual in a
single state of disturbance.

Minimum dose also refers to appropriate repetition
of doses. In Paragraphs 246 and 247 of the *Organon,*

Hahnemann makes it clear that the remedy should be repeated only when the vital force clearly indicates the need for more medicine and then in slightly modified potency, because the former dose has already accomplished the expected change in the vital force, therefore a second, dynamically unchanged dose of the same medicine no longer finds the vital force in the same condition or state of susceptibility as it was before.

When it comes to second prescription progress assessment, it would be impossible to perceive accurately what had happened to the patient and why, if several different medicines, in several different potencies had been administered.

Direction of Cure

This principle comes into play as we observe nature's distinct curative pattern. Individuals recover from illness by throwing off disease in a particular direction.

Symptoms appear and disappear from above to below, from within to without, in the reverse order of their appearance, the most recent symptoms disappear first, and symptoms experienced longest disappear last, (and, according to some classical homoeopaths, via the shortest, safest route). The principle of Direction of Cure forms a substantial part of second prescription deliberations. After a remedy has been given, the homoeopath closely scrutinizes the directional movement of the patient's symptoms to decide if the remedy response is curative or not.

Herbert Roberts gave a clear description of the law of Direction of Cure in his *Principles and Art of Cure by Homoeopathy:*

> Under a cure, the symptoms of a deranged vital function always disappear in the reverse order of their appearance. This is true in acute as well as chronic disturbances. Because this order is always maintained it is a vital point of observation in taking the case to note the sequence of symptoms in invasion, so that the physician can know of the progress of the case under the selected remedy. In very serious cases, when we are so anxious to know what improvement is taking place, we can be assured by watching the order of the disappearance of the symptoms. In this way we can learn the action of the remedy in its assistance to the vital force and can give an accurate prognosis. This is equally true in acute or chronic states.[7]

Improvement and cure come from within outward. Just as no growth and development can take place from outside inward, so no hope of cure can be held that moves in a contrary direction. Growth and development and cure are centrifugal and never centripetal.[8]

Symptoms disappear from above downward; complaints go from an important organ to a less important organ; symptoms disappear in the reverse order of their appearance.[9]

One of the best illustrations is the rheumatic fever manifestation. This is a case where the joints of the extremities are first attacked, next the joints nearer the body, and presently we find the heart involved. This is the natural order of the onset of the symptoms. Now if we relieve the symptoms appearing in the extremities, are we approaching a cure? Consider the vital organs that are in danger, if they are not already attacked. But under the exhibition of the carefully selected homoeopathic remedy the more important organs are the first to be freed (being the last organs to be attacked) and gradually the manifestations recede to the extremities, the first to be attacked.[10]

Understanding Direction of Cure is critically important in second prescription. It prevents many unnecessary mistakes and provides a useful evaluation base.

Totality

Understanding and application of the above eight principles in their entirety will enhance the effectiveness of any homoeopathic practitioner. But without understanding and application of the principle of Totality, the most effective prescribing is beyond reach. As Kent puts it:

The success of prescribing depends upon the view taken of the totality of the symptoms.

To be able to view the totality of symptoms so that the most similar remedy will appear to the mind is the aim of all healing artists. As the view varies, so varies the success.[11]

Currently many homoeopaths view disordered individuals from a wide variety of perspectives. Some practitioners view cases from the pathological aspect; others view the patient's temperament, color of eyes, hair. Others take the astrological or numerological view of patients. Still others view cases through keynote symptoms or solely in the light of miasms. Another tendency is to view patients solely from a psychoanalytical perspective. Each of these perspectives views individuals in part, but not as a whole; at best they form a partial and yet somewhat distorted view of the case. None of them relate to the true *totality* view.

Totality as a method of case analysis is often misunderstood. It doesn't mean compiling a long list of all the symptoms and arriving at a numerical match with a given remedy.

> The totality, in homoeopathic practice, is the true diagnosis of the disease, and at the same time the diagnosis of the remedy. The totality eliminates all the theoretical elements and the speculations of traditional medicine and deals only with the actually manifest facts. The facts it assembles, not according to some arbitrary or imaginary form, but according to a natural order.[12]

Hahnemann mentions the principle of Totality throughout the *Organon,* and clearly defines it in Paragraph 7:

the totality of these symptoms, *of this out-
rdly reflected picture of the internal essence
ᴗ, the disease, that is, of the affection of the vital force,* must be the principal, or the sole
means, whereby the disease can make known
what remedy it requires—the only thing that
can determine the choice of the most appropriate remedy—and thus in a word the totality of
symptoms must be the principal, indeed the
only thing the physician has to take note of in
every case of the disease and to remove by
means of his art, in order that the disease shall
be cured and transformed into health.[13]

In the footnote to this paragraph, Hahnemann
carefully illustrates the issue of viewing the individual in
less than the totality, which he says results is a *one-sided*
procedure:

A single one of the symptoms present is no
more the disease itself than a single foot is the
man himself.[14]

In the *Organon,* Paragraphs 15 through 19, Hahnemann makes it clear that we must recognize that the totality of the disease symptoms and the disease itself are
one and the same thing. And in Paragraph 153 Hahnemann tells us how to perceive the appropriate symptoms to arrive at the portrait of the individual's totality
of suffering. He says we must be guided to the single
correct medicine for each individual by noting the more
striking, singular, uncommon, and peculiar (characteristic) signs and symptoms. *The strange, rare, and peculiar*

concomitant, modifying, sensation and affinity symptoms form the unique blueprint of the individual's disturbed state. This corresponds to the symptom image totality of the appropriate medicine documented in the materia medica.

When such a perfect undistorted view of the whole mental, physical, emotional totality presents itself to the unprejudiced, observing, perceiving practitioner, the prescription becomes easy. Homoeopathy is the medicine of individualization.

> Really the totality is simply the complete picture of the disease. The totality is to the disease what the man, the ego, is to his organism. It is that which gives individuality and personality.[15]

> The totality is related equally to the remedy and to the disease. They are counterparts; they may even be considered as identical as to origin and nature in the last analysis.[16]

> When all the symptoms of a case have been gathered, and the totality has been found, we have all that can be known of the disease.[17]

Totality of symptoms leads directly to the individuality of the disturbance and therefore directly to the remedy that fits that particular state of disorder and, ultimately, to cure according to the Law of Similars. Here it's worth mentioning a diagrammatic representation of totality derived from the work of Boenninghausen and Hering among others:

THE SYMPTOM IMAGE TOTALITY

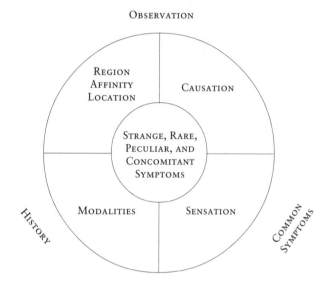

OBSERVATION

REGION
AFFINITY
LOCATION

CAUSATION

STRANGE, RARE,
PECULIAR, AND
CONCOMITANT
SYMPTOMS

MODALITIES   SENSATION

HISTORY

COMMON
SYMPTOMS

TOTALITY = INDIVIDUALITY, PERSONALITY
OF
SICKNESS AND MEDICINE

Understanding Hahnemann's principles enables us to resolve dilemmas facing us during the second prescription phase, for they tell us how to make sense of the case. As Kent cautions:

> If he is not conversant with the import of what he sees, he will undertake to do wrong things, he will make wrong prescriptions, he will change his medicines and do things to the detriment of the patient.[18]

Understanding the import of what one *sees* means understanding the natural laws that govern the practice of classical homoeopathy. Take a moment to review them and you will find that it is ultimately these clearly comprehensible principles which teach us how to perceive both the disordered state of the patient and the way to restoration of order and health. As I said earlier, these codes of practice are all to be found in the *Organon*. It is their thoughtful application that enables practitioners to successfully fulfill Hahnemann's job description for homoeopaths, laid out in Paragraphs 3 and 4 of the *Organon:*

> If the physician clearly perceives what is to be cured in diseases, that is to say, in every individual case of disease (*knowledge of disease, indication*), if he clearly perceives what is curative in medicines, that is to say, in each individual medicine (*knowledge of medicinal powers*), and if he knows how to adapt, according to clearly defined principles, what is curative in medicines to what he has discovered to be undoubtedly morbid in the patient, so that the recovery must ensue to adapt it, as well in respect to the suitability of the medicine most appropriate according to its mode of action to the case before him (*choice of the remedy, the medicine indicated*), as also in respect to the exact mode of preparation and quantity of it required (*proper dose*), and the proper period for repeating the dose; if, finally, he knows the obstacles to recovery in each case and is aware how to remove them, so that the restoration may be permanent, *then he understands how to*

treat judiciously and rationally, and he is a true practitioner of the healing art . . . He is likewise a preserver of health if he knows the things that derange health and cause disease, and how to remove them from persons in health.[19]

CHAPTER 1

1. Kent, *Lectures on Homoeopathic Philosophy,* Chapter 1.
2. Hahnemann, *Organon,* 6th ed. (Boericke trans.), ¶9.
3. Hahnemann, *Organon,* 6th ed. (Wesselhoeft trans.), ¶26, 27.
4. Hahnemann, *Organon,* 6th ed. (Boericke trans.), Preface, pg. 18.
5. Hahnemann, *Organon,* 6th ed. (Boericke trans.), ¶273.
6. Hahnemann, *Organon,* 6th ed. (Boericke trans.), Preface, pg. 19.
7. Roberts, *The Principles and Art of Cure by Homoeopathy,* Chapter 4, pg. 44–45.
8. Roberts, *The Principles and Art of Cure by Homoeopathy,* Chapter 4, pg. 44–45.
9. Roberts, *The Principles and Art of Cure by Homoeopathy,* Chapter 4, pg. 44–45.
10. Roberts, *The Principles and Art of Cure by Homoeopathy,* Chapter 4, pg. 44–45.
11. Kent, *Minor Writings, The View of Successful Prescribing,* pg. 642.
12. Boenninghausen, *Therapeutic Pocketbook,* Introduction by H.A. Roberts, pg. 16.
13. Hahnemann, *Organon,* 6th ed. (Boericke trans.), ¶7.

14. Hahnemann, *Organon,* 6th ed. (Boericke trans.),
    Footnote 4, ¶7.

15. Boenninghausen, *Therapeutic Pocketbook,*
    Introduction by H.A. Roberts / Annie C. Wilson,
    pg. 11.

16. Boenninghausen, *Therapeutic Pocketbook,*
    Introduction by H.A. Roberts / Annie C. Wilson,
    pg. 13.

17. Boenninghausen, *Therapeutic Pocketbook,*
    Introduction by H.A. Roberts / Annie C. Wilson,
    pg. 15.

18. Kent, *Lectures on Homoeopathic Philosophy,*
    Lecture 35, pg. 224.

19. Hahnemann, *Organon,* 6th ed. (Boericke trans.), ¶3.

CHAPTER 2

The Second Prescription—
Demanding, Suspenseful, Rewarding

THE SECOND PRESCRIPTION STAGE is thrilling because
it is the point at which homoeopaths flex the mind
muscle, sharpen the intellect, and demonstrate their
keenly attuned detective skills. It is the moment where
we employ our considerable powers of *observation* and
analysis to the fullest, and if all is going according to
plan, second prescription is the climax of job satisfac-
tion.[1]

The evaluation, analysis, and decision-making process involved in the homoeopathic second prescription
must also be the most challenging, suspenseful, and rewarding aspect of homoeopathic practice. There is a
great deal at stake—the patient's restored well being,
continued suffering, or decline.

What Exactly Is the Second Prescription?

Strictly speaking, according to Kent, the second
prescription is the prognosis after observing the action
of the remedy that has worked.[2]

At the second prescription stage, the patient has
had the first prescription and we are waiting for the reaction of the vital force to display itself. This is the mo-

ment we've been waiting for, the moment patient and practitioner should observe the curative power of homoeopathy. We are on the edge of our seats with suspense waiting to see how close we came to matching the remedy to the symptom image totality. Within minutes in acute treatment, hours, days or weeks in chronic treatment, the patient's response to the first prescription indicates the beginning of gentle, rapid restoration of health or continued decline. If cure has begun, we glimpse the exciting possibility of the individual fulfilling full mental, emotional, and physical potential.

Now is the time we see homoeopathy at work, because the patient's response to the first prescription confounds skeptics who say homoeopathy is merely placebo effect. Although placebo may produce general improvement, patients mostly describe placebo effects in diffuse, vague terms. By contrast, patients responding to the action of homoeopathic medicines clearly describe a definite improvement or worsening of symptoms reflected in their disease picture and their medical history. More importantly, placebo rarely, if ever, produces a return of old symptoms previously experienced in the patient's medical history. To the eagle-eyed homoeopath, the return of historical symptoms indicates the degree to which the curative power of the vital force has been triggered, and whether the patient is going in the right (curative) or wrong direction. It's especially satisfying when the patient reports return of a symptom she forgot she had in the past, and didn't tell you about in the history taking. Why? Because it directly confounds the theory that homoeopathy is just placebo effect.

In the second prescription phase we need to determine, on every level of the patient's being, if and to
what degree the individual is under the power of the homoeopathic medicine. To do this we need to exercise
objectivity, critical thinking, and meticulous attention
to detail.

> After administration of the simillimum some
> action should result. It is upon our interpreta-
> tion of the remedy action (or the reaction of the
> vital force to the remedy) that a successful sec-
> ond prescription largely depends.[3]

As we follow the case, we must track the activity
and state of the vital force by thoroughly checking the
reactions of the patient in the context of the original,
presenting case.

As stated earlier, in homoeopathy, symptoms serve
several critically important purposes. The only way the
vital force is visible to the human eye is through its expression of symptoms, which are the distress signals of
the vital force. In the natural curative process as best as
it is able, the human organism vents the inner imbalance or disturbance centrifugally, away from the vital
organs of the body through symptoms. This means at
any moment the strength or weakness of the organism is
largely unknown except through symptoms. After the
patient takes a remedy, depending on the accuracy or
inaccuracy of the first prescription, the symptoms begin
to change for better or worse according to the Direction
of Cure.

The great challenge of the second prescription lies
in confirming that the first prescription acted, under-

standing how and why it acted or didn't act, and deciding with confidence what to do next. By comparison,
the decision-making complexity of the second prescription process makes the first prescription look remark-
ably easy yet most of us know how difficult that can be!

Being human, homoeopaths make mistakes. To be
successful, the important thing is to spot the errors and
correct them as quickly as possible.

> It pays to be careful and "go slow" in the be-
> ginning; then there will not be so many mis-
> takes to correct. We should examine our case
> carefully and systematically, select our first
> remedy and potency with care, give our first
> dose, if the single dose is decided upon and
> then watch results. If the remedy and dose are
> right *there will be results*. We need have no
> doubt on that score. The indicated remedy and
> potency, even in a single dose cannot be given
> without some result and the result must be
> good.[4]

During the follow-up and second prescription
phase, a peculiar interdependence between the practitioner and the patient's symptoms prevails.

> After a prescription has been made the physi-
> cian commences to make observations. The
> whole future of the patient may depend upon
> the conclusions that the physician arrives at
> from these observations, for his action depends
> very much upon his observations, and upon his
> action depends the good of the patient.[5]

Subsequent actions depend on intelligent interpretation of careful observations.

> After we have selected what we believe to be the indicated remedy and administered it in proper potency and dosage, it is our duty to observe the patient carefully in order that we may correctly note and intelligently interpret the changes that occur; for upon these changes in the patient's condition, as revealed by the symptoms, depends our subsequent action in the further treatment of the case.[6]

It is at this critical moment in the patient's improving or declining state of health that he arrives at a crossroads to cure. There is a natural eagerness to hasten cure. Nevertheless, allowing ourselves to be overwhelmed by enthusiasm to fix things fast or jumping to the wrong conclusions about what has happened is all it takes to interrupt the curative response and spoil a good preceding prescription, confusing cases by too early or too frequent remedy repetition or changing remedies too soon. The natural, curative momentum of the vital force towards cure takes time and goes at its own, individual pace. It is foolhardy to try to hurry the vital force along, because of patient pressure or practitioner impatience, for some action or response within a certain time frame. It is very important that we observe and pace our actions strictly according to the pace of the vital force. In this way patient and practitioner reap the reward of rapid cure.

As well as integrity and unbounded patience, the necessary essential skills for a successful second prescription are acute perception, rigorous observation, focused concentration, and attentive listening, along with meticulous accuracy of data collection and record keeping.

If the homoeopathic physician is not an accurate observer, his observations will be indefinite; and if his observations are indefinite, his prescribing is indefinite.[7]

The accurate homoeopathic second prescription relies on the practitioner's clarity in evaluating the curative, suppressive, palliative, or ineffectual results of the first prescription based on the quality of patient information received. Meticulously checking through the mental, emotional, and physical symptoms, we note every significant detail. Our detective skills honed to perfection, we perceive that the central disturbance is eradicated or the individual is moving in a curative direction, and if, and to what degree, the patient remains under the power of the homoeopathic medicine.

It is important to approach the follow-up with an open mind, free of hopes or attachment to the success of your first prescription. To be successful, homoeopaths must develop a healthy, self-critical attitude and the highest degree of diligence and integrity.

In this most complex patient evaluation process we strive to develop that wonderful, objective state Hahnemann calls *the unprejudiced observer,* freedom from bias and prejudice on any level. Cultivating and maintaining the unprejudiced observer state is very difficult, but I believe it is the key to effective homoeopathy because it enables us to listen attentively to the patient and observe those critically important, characteristic symptoms upon which all prescriptions are based. In practical terms, this means leaving our personal "baggage," likes and dislikes, value systems, as well as preconceptions of patients and remedies, outside the interview room and far away from the case, lest they inadvertently prejudice our case management and analysis. As Hahnemann cautions us in Paragraph 6 of the *Organon,* the unprejudiced observer is well aware of the futility of transcendental speculation. The impact upon our patients of setting aside the ego and resurrecting that rare human quality, humility, is extremely powerful and curative.

In order to obtain clear definite evidence, we must educate the patient from the first interview, making it clear that, in contrast to dominant medical practice, in the homoeopathic healing process seemingly insignificant changes on mental, physical, and emotional levels may signal important effects of the homoeopathic medicine.

> It is for us to determine what the reaction means and to interpret it in prognostic terms.[8]

> We must discriminate between that which is reaction and that which calls for a remedy.[9]

In evaluating the patient's improvement or decline, we look at the patient's total response to the medicine, seeking to know precisely where the changes have occurred, and what is the degree and nature of the change. The patient's ability or inability to respond to the medicine, the disappearance of symptoms, the return of old symptoms, and the degree of amelioration or aggravation tell us the action or inaction of the remedy on the vital force.

We must be able to listen to the patient's report and from it and our powers of observation to determine what the remedy is doing.[10]

What Can We Expect to Happen?

If the remedy and dosage are accurately and homoeopathically selected, according to the state of the patient's vital force, susceptibility, and predominant miasms, the homoeopathic medicine stimulates the body's defense mechanism to heal the organism in its uniquely individual way.

In the typical curative homoeopathic response to the remedy, the vital force is stimulated to gradually exteriorize the inner disturbance according to nature's Direction of Cure. This occurs from above down, from within to without, from more vital to less vital organs, and in reverse chronological order. The responses to centesimal and LM potencies differ. The response evaluations that follow all refer to the centesimal potencies. (LM criteria are explained in Chapter 5.)

During the initial stage of the curative process, soon after the medicinal potencies are administered, the remedy typically causes a slight, fleeting, perhaps imperceptible intensification of the *original, existing, characteristic symptoms*. This quickly subsides. At the same time the patient feels much better in herself.

The true homoeopathic aggravation, I say, is when the symptoms are worse, but the patient says, "I feel better."[11]

On the other hand, if the selection of remedy and potency are inaccurate there may be no reaction at all, or the individual grows worse in herself and the *disease symptoms* become aggravated and more intense. Obviously this situation indicates a non-curative, unfavorable response to the action of the medicine.

Evaluating Remedy Response

One of the biggest problems in homoeopathic practice is correct evaluation of remedy response. Success hinges on this evaluation, so from material researched, I have endeavored to create clear and specific guidelines for the follow-up interview. Of course, each practitioner will bring her own understanding to the evaluation process, but remembering these important points can make all the difference between success or failure.

In order to accurately evaluate the action of the remedy, we must ask the right kind of questions and make the most accurate possible comparison of the case before and after the remedy was taken. Begin by asking *yourself* these questions:

• Since the patient took the medicine, what exactly did happen? ("The facts, ma'am, just the facts.")

• Did the remedy act? How can I be sure something really happened? Is the remedy still acting? What demonstrable evidence do I have?

• Has the patient's state of vital force changed, become stronger or weaker, and to what degree? How do I know this?

• Have the characteristic, distinguishing, individualizing symptoms of the patient or the pathognomonic (common to the disease) symptoms changed?

• Is the patient truly better, the same, or worse? Once again, what evidence do I have to support this assessment?

• What is the correct expected curative response? Does the patient's response fit the homoeopathic model of cure?

• Was the first medicine the exact simillimum prescription, or does the patient's response indicate a partially acting remedy that didn't complete the cure because it reflected only part of the symptom image totality? How do I know which it is?

• Was the first prescription curative, palliative, or suppressive, and what is the evidence? (Although the terms curative and palliative are easily understood, the term suppression may not be. Once again, by delving into *Webster's* dictionary, our understanding begins— "Medical suppression: the complete stoppage of a natural secretion or excretion, suppressed urine." The homoeopathic curative process safely encourages and promotes the natural, curative secretion, excretion, exteriorization, or expression of disorder. In homoeopathy we understand that in a state of imbalance, natural processes are often increased as the body's self-healing mechanism, unaided, attempts to vent and exteriorize the innermost disturbance. Correct selection of the homoeopathic medicine harnesses and expedites the natural expression of disorder in order to release the organism of burdensome symptoms and rapidly reestablish equilibrium throughout the whole person.)

- What should I do next?
- Do I need to repeat the remedy, and why?
- Do I give the same or a different potency, and why?
- Is a different remedy required? Why is it needed? What should it be? What should the potency be, and why?

In a chronic case, the patient generally makes a progress report about a month after taking the first remedy.* This examination is different from but just as methodical and thorough as the initial intake. The following section discusses in detail how to elicit appropriate information.

As in the initial case taking, the best, clearest information for case study comes from asking open-ended questions that invite patients to think deeply about their answers. Voluntered, unprompted, spontaneous information is the most valuable of all. Asking open-ended questions avoids committing the unforgivable sin of putting words in the patient's mouth, thereby risking inaccuracy and confusion. As in the initial intake interview, always ask for specific examples of any changes the patient experienced. Indefinite answers like "I feel

---

* LM follow-ups occur more frequently. See Chapter 5.

fine, everything is OK," or "I'm in a bad way," or "I feel worse," are useless for case assessment purposes because they tell us nothing specific about the patient's state. Also, disconcertingly, patients will often say they feel better because they so much want to get well and have great faith in homoeopathic treatment.

To avoid inaccurate interpretations and ensure the truth of information received, so as to make as accurate an evaluation of the patient's current state as possible, we must always ask: "In what way are things fine? Give me an example."

As much as possible it is best to let the patient tell the story of her present state and reaction to the remedy, without too much interference from questions. However, open questions are often needed to fill out the details. Often when patients are better they don't notice the disappearance of specific symptoms because their attention is now free to be directed elsewhere. Always remember, it's essential that you know *why* you are asking each question. In other words what kind of information do you seek from a particular line of inquiry?

Below are typical questions you could ask if necessary to help patients report responses to remedies. Obviously the data sought will differ slightly depending on the acute or chronic nature of the disorder you are being consulted about. Many of the following questions are geared to chronic cases. The patient's answer will determine whether there has been a change, what has changed, the degree the symptoms have changed, and the direction the disorder is going. It will indicate whether the patient is the same, better, or worse.

1. What happened during the first few days after you took the remedy? What did you experience during the first few days and weeks? What changes occurred in that time?

By asking this we want to know whether there was a perceived initial reaction to the medicine. The answer indicates the patient's positive, negative, or nonexistent response and likewise the perceptible reaction of the vital force to the action of the homoeopathic medicine.

2. How are the symptoms you originally complained about? Have they changed in any way? Are they better or worse? In what way have they changed?

We need to know the specific changes and pattern of change since the last interview. It is important to actually refer to your original case notes to compare them with the current report. For pain symptoms, the 0–10 scale is a useful comparison. A patient who has been in pain for years may not actually notice a change of degree in the pain until questioned this way. The pattern of change during the month following administration of the remedy will indicate the degree of progress or decline.

3. How have you managed the stresses in your life? Have there been any significant changes at home or work, with the family, or partner?

We want to know if there has been a change in the patient's ability to adapt to changes in his life. The answer to this question reveals possible changes in an individual's ability to manage stresses in life's circumstances. After all, health is successful adaptation.

> 4. *Have there been any changes in your feelings, needs, your ability to think, concentrate, or focus; in your memory; loves, fears, anxieties, aversions, longings, experience of feelings, emotions?*

The answer to these kinds of questions is extremely important because they elicit information about changes in a patient's mental/emotional state, the innermost state of the person. We want to know if there are any differences in the way the patient manages or experiences emotion, levels or causation of anxieties, the surfacing or internalizing of new or old feelings. For example, in response to the first medicine, we may see an individual who was silent, cut off, and shut down before the medicine, become more open, lively, active, or talkative after it. Or the individual wept only when alone before treatment and now cries openly; or a sad and depressed individual before, is now lighthearted, happier, joking, smiling, and laughing more. Be especially alert to this answer. Alternately, we could see all this in reverse. If the answer indicates a worsening of the mental/emotional state, ask:

> 5. *Did anything happen recently that might have caused this response?*

This question determines whether an exciting or maintaining cause such as shock, trauma, injury, aggravation of a particular situation, or activation of an underlying miasm is responsible for this symptom shift and not the action of our ill-selected remedy. It's important to know the difference; otherwise we risk changing the original medicine at the wrong time and ultimately muddling up the case. To ensure clarity of understanding the individual's answer to this question, determine whether or not this is the usual response to such situations or a different response, indicating a specific course of action to be taken. Check back through your original case notes to be sure that this is not a return of an old disordered state that was only temporarily relieved or suppressed in the past by medication or other means. For information about what action to take in a deteriorating mental situation see Chapter 4.

> 6. *How is your sleep now compared with before the remedy? How do you feel when you wake? Give examples of any changes.*

In sleep the brain's activity changes. Sleep is a change of state from outer conscious to inner unconscious states. The answer to this question is important because it will reveal aspects of the innermost and be a useful guide to what is going on in the patient at a deep level. Ideally, the sleep pattern should satisfy our need for rest and we should awaken refreshed.

> 7. *Overall, how has your energy/vitality/motivation been affected since the remedy? To what degree? Can you give examples of any change experienced at any level to any degree?*

We want to see whether there has been an upward or downward energy shift, and to what degree. This answer gives us important information on the state of the vital force and the state of the individual's innermost will, understanding, and intellect. In health, we have good energy and feel motivated to do things. Compare states before and after the remedy. Use the 0–10 scale if you find it useful. Specific examples of changes are very important; don't settle for vague information, as it will mislead you.

> 8. *Has there been any change in the way you respond to things that affect you generally as a whole? For example, changes in temperature, responses to the weather, days of the month, or time of year.*

This answer reveals any changes in the individual as a whole. Perhaps before he was deeply affected by weather changes, which induced headaches, and now he can experience changes of weather without getting a headache.

> 9. *For women—How were you before, during, and after your last period?*

Another extremely important question, because the answer concerns a discharge from inside the organism, telling us something about the innermost workings and state of the vital force. Depending on the individual concerned, before, after, and during menstruation, women can be affected on all levels, mentally and emotionally as well as physically. According to Kent, blood relates to love.[12] Because our loves are of the innermost, because the menstrual cycle is such a significant part of a woman's being, the state of the menstrual cycle reflects the innermost state of the person. The answer to this question will give us a particularly good idea of what's happening to the individual as a whole, and it will be included in the symptom image totality.

10. Have you experienced any new symptoms you've never, ever had before?

The appearance of new symptoms always worries patients and practitioners, so the answer to this question is especially significant as it relates to whether or not the medicine was correct or incorrect in nature or dosage. If the patient reports *new* symptoms, confirm that this is true because it is an *unfavorable* sign. To ascertain if new symptoms are definitely new, scan your chronology of symptoms thoroughly to check whether the symptom described is actually an *old* symptom that the patient forgot she had because it disappeared long ago. Or perhaps the "new" symptom is a symptom the patient has become used to over time, but because of its recent increased intensity she is more aware of it and has become concerned about it. A detailed discussion of the appearance of new symptoms and appropriate action to be taken is provided in Chapter 4.

Having asked these or similar questions of your own, allow the patient to elaborate on each answer, check through the case notes again carefully and ask for a symptom-by-symptom report. Before ending the interview make sure you understand all the changes that have occurred and you've noted any prominent or subtle stabilization, destabilization, improvement, or decline in the patient's state. It is essential, for successful prescribing, to observe any strengthening or weakening of the condition. Subtle changes may be imperceptible to the patient, but the practitioner must be able to perceive them, to ensure that the correct momentum and Direction of Cure is sustained. Close puts it most succinctly:

> In deciding the question whether the remedy has acted or not, we must be careful not to be misled by the opinions or prejudices of the patient or his attendants. Some patients, having all their interest and attention centered upon some particular symptom which they regard as all-important, will assert that there has been no change; that they are no better, or even worse than they were before they took the remedy. These statements should be received with great caution and we should proceed to go over the symptom-record item by item with care. We need not antagonize the patient by gruffly asserting that he must be mistaken, but may express our regret or sympathy and then quietly question him as to each particular symptom. We will frequently find that the patient has really improved in many important respects, although the pet symptom (often constipation) is as yet unchanged.[13]

In the patient progress interview, just as in the original case taking, always check the detail of what the patient reports. Always ask for concrete examples. Before taking any action, ask yourself why you are doing what you are doing and what solid evidence you have for a particular action. In other words, what specific principles of practice have you applied in the evaluation of the patient in the current state following the first prescription?

Records to the Rescue

As homoeopaths, we have a tendency to strive for perfection in our work because we understand that avoidance of errors is crucial, as much for the well-being of the patient as for the reputation of homoeopathy. However, homoeopaths are only human. So no matter how hard we try not to, we are bound to make all kinds of errors for all kinds of reasons. In addition to good training, the best way to minimize mistakes is to thoroughly record your case taking and case analysis. If the complete decision-making process is briefly but clearly documented in the patient's file, looking back through a properly recorded case, the practitioner can quickly locate and rectify mistakes. As Kent tells patients:

> You should have no confidence in the experience of men who do not write out faithfully all the symptoms of the patient treated, and note carefully the remedy, and how given. Especially is this necessary in patients likely to need a second prescription . . . Homoeopathy is nothing if not true and, if true, the greatest accuracy of detail and method should be followed.[14]

A busy practice means it's difficult to clearly recall each patient's previous state. To accurately and quickly assess patient progress and avoid relying solely on possibly malfunctioning memory, I find it extremely useful to plot patient response on a progress chart. This gives me an easily accessible reference guide to the direction the patient and pathology are going. Custom-make your own and you'll have an at-a-glance, instant image of what was happening the last time the patient communicated with you, which can be easily compared to the current state.

Common sense dictates when the unexpected telephone call comes, don't grab the nearest notebook or scrap of paper to jot down patient comments. You may forget to file the notes, or worse still, mislay them. It's best to never ask or write anything until the patient's file is in front of you. A much more precise and accurate evaluation occurs if all patient responses are documented in the file, with the date and time of the communication clearly recorded. The progress chart is particularly valuable when the patient contacts you in an emergency. Well-kept case records can be a real lifesaver in a busy practice.

CHAPTER 2

1. Kent, *Lectures on Homoeopathic Philosophy,* Lecture 36.
2. Kent, *Lectures on Homoeopathic Philosophy,* Lecture 35.
3. Roberts, *The Principles and Art of Cure by Homoeopathy,* Chapter 9.
4. Close, *The Genius of Homoeopathy,* Chapter 13, pg. 203.
5. Kent, *Lectures on Homoeopathic Philosophy,* Lecture 35, pg. 224.
6. Close, *The Genius of Homoeopathy,* Chapter 13, pg. 205.

7. Kent, *Lectures on Homoeopathic Philosophy*, Lecture 35, pg. 224.

8. Roberts, *The Principles and Art of Cure by Homoeopathy*, Chapter 14, pg. 124.

9. Kent, *Lectures on Homoeopathic Philosophy*, Lecture 34, pg. 216.

10. Roberts, *The Principles and Art of Cure by Homoeopathy*, Chapter 14, pg. 124.

11. Kent, *Lectures on Homoeopathic Philosophy*, Lecture 35.

12. Kent, *Minor Writings*, pg. 601.

13. Close, *The Genius of Homoeopathy*, Chapter 13, pg. 205.

14. Kent, *Minor Writings*, pg. 239.

CHAPTER 3

What to Look For at the Follow-Up

IN THE PREVIOUS CHAPTER we discussed an effective method of examining the patient in order to elicit information about possible changes in mental, physical, and emotional states arising from the action of a remedy.

> After we have selected what we believe to be the indicated remedy and administered it in proper potency and dosage, it is our duty to observe the patient carefully in order that we may correctly note and intelligently interpret the changes that occur; for upon these changes in the patient's condition, as revealed by the symptoms, depends our subsequent action in the further treatment of the case.[1]

The changes that have occurred will tell us whether the remedy acted or not, the scope, effect, and depth of its action, and if it didn't act why it didn't and what to do next.

How Remedies Act

If we are to select the correct remedy, potency, and dosage at both first and second prescription stages of treatment, we must first of all understand how homoeopathic medicines act in the body. As Kent said:

The object of the first prescription is to arrange the vital current or motion in a direction favorable to equilibrium . . .[2]

In other words, the aim is to bring about cure and restore balance in the individual. In the *Organon*, Hahnemann said we are more susceptible to medicines than disease causing agents:

. . . it is undeniably shown by all experience that the living human organism is much more disposed and has a greater liability to be acted on, and to have its health deranged by medicinal powers, than by morbific noxious agents . . . medicinal agents have an absolute unconditional power, greatly superior to [morbific agents].[3]

In *Chronic Diseases* Hahnemann succinctly describes how homoeopathic medicines act.

. . . if the image of the morbific foe be magnified to the apprehension of the vital principle through homoeopathic medicines, which . . . simulate the original disease, we gradually cause and compel this instinctive vital force to increase its energies by degrees . . . and at last to such a degree that it becomes far more powerful than the original disease. The consequence of this is, that the vital force again becomes sovereign in its domain, can again hold and direct the reins of sanitary progress, while the apparent increase of the disease caused by homoeopathic medicines, disappears of itself . . .[4]

On the basis of the Law of Similars, remedies act by simulating the dynamic quality of the natural disease and the vital force. This process only occurs if the dynamic quality of the medicine matches the totality of the individual's presenting symptom image. To act curatively the remedy must not only be similar in symptom-causing potential, it must also be a little stronger than the individual's natural disease. This is achieved by selecting the attenuated dynamized potency that best matches the strength or weakness of the individual's vital force.

After lengthy experimentation, Hahnemann was the first to observe the duality of drug action on the living organism.[5] He perceived that every medicine and every stimulus has the power to act upon or affect life, and by degree deranges, disturbs the life force, producing certain changes that last for a longer or shorter time. Through the drug provings, Hahnemann observed that any drug administered to sick or healthy people, no matter the dosage, gives rise to two events: (1) altered states; (2) a succession of symptom patterns.

The first symptom-pattern Hahnemann termed the *primary action* or immediate action of the drug on the organism. At this point the life preserving vital force submits to the influence of the power acting on it from outside and allows itself to be modified by it.

This is followed by the second symptom pattern, which Hahnemann termed *secondary* action symptoms, which symptoms are the organism's reaction to the primary drug effects and are more or less opposite to them.

Having discovered this dual action of drugs, Hahnemann concluded that if the primary effect symptoms of the homoeopathic drug on healthy individuals were similar to but stronger than the symptoms of a sick person, the organism's secondary reactive symptoms would act to remove the sick person's symptoms and restore health. Through these observations, Hahnemann arrived at the homoeopathic application of the Law of Similars.

As a result of Hahnemann's experiments and observations, we understand how homoeopathic medicines act by stimulating a secondary, defensive, compensatory, and curative reaction of the organism to the disturbance-causing stimulus. Therefore, administration of homoeopathic medicines strengthens and supports the body's defensive reaction.

Having understood how homoeopathic medicine works, the next step demands that we determine:

Has the Remedy Acted or Not?

Homoeopaths rarely take anything for granted. We thoughtfully and consistently ask ourselves what evidence is there that a particular remedy acted. As Close says:

A remedy shows its action: (1) by producing new symptoms; (2) by the disappearance of symptoms; (3) by the increase or aggravation of symptoms; (4) by the amelioration of symptoms; (5) by a change in the order and direction of symptoms.[6]

The action of the remedy is shown by changes in the nature, location, and quality of both *characteristic* and *pathognomonic* symptoms experienced by the patient, as observed and recorded by the practitioner. These changes reflect the state of the vital force after the remedy. The next action depends upon the character of the changes. All changes must be carefully studied and evaluated.

> Now, if a medicine acts it commences immediately to effect changes in the patient, and these changes are shown by signs and symptoms. The inner nature of the disease appears to the physician through the symptoms, and it is like watching the hands upon the clock. This watching and waiting and observing has to be done by the physician in order that he may judge by the changes what to do, and what not to do . . . There is always an index that tells him what not to do. If he is a sharp and vigilant observer he will see the index for every case.[7]

What is this index or reliable evidence of the remedy's action?

> We have in the symptoms that which we can rely upon . . . The symptoms themselves must be corroborated. The patient's opinion must be corroborated by the symptoms. The symptoms do corroborate what the patient says in many instances, but the symptoms are the physician's most satisfactory evidence.[8]

How may we accurately differentiate between the different changes that can occur?

> Make a difference in your mind between organic changes that take place in the organs that

are vital, that carry on the work of the economy, and organic changes that take place in structures of the body that are not essential to life.[9]

The aim of homoeopathy is eradication of the innermost causation, the central disturbance of the disease, and complete restoration of health. How can we know the patient will recover?

> . . . we should know by the symptoms if the changes occurring are sufficiently interior . . . Incurable diseases will very often be palliated by mild medicines that act only superficially, act upon the sensorium, act upon the senses, and, though the hidden and deep-seated trouble goes on and progresses, and is sometimes made worse, yet the patient is made comfortable. So that by the symptoms we can know whether the changes that are occurring are of sufficient depth, so that the patient may recover.[10]

In observing patient responses, we need to distinguish between changes occurring in vital organs and changes in superficial tissues and nonvital organs. This means we must look for the *Direction of Cure.*

In the symptom timeline, look for an *orderly* or *disorderly change of direction.* Examine carefully the degree of symptom intensity increase, decrease, or no change. Always look at the location of symptoms to determine their direction. Are they proceeding correctly from mental plane to physical plane, or incorrectly, vice versa? Next, pay careful attention to any shifts in whatever exciting, maintaining, or fundamental causation is uppermost in the case. It may happen that an exciting cause becomes a maintaining cause, e.g. an unresolved injury, or the activity of the underlying predisposition (miasm) changes.

Determining whether the action of medicines is curative, suppressive, or palliative requires us to know why some symptoms disappear and others reappear. Close reminds us:

> The Direction of Cure is from within outward, from above downward, and in the reverse order of the appearance of the symptoms. By this test we may always know whether we are curing or only palliating a disease. The last appearing symptoms of a disease should be the first to disappear under the action of a curative remedy.[11]

Close gives the following example of the correct Direction of Cure:

> When old skin eruptions reappear, old ulcers break out again, old fistulae reopen, old discharges flow again, swollen tubercular glands become inflamed, break down, and suppurate away; old joint pains return; the patient's heart, lung, kidney, liver, spleen, or brain symptoms in the meantime *improving* then we know that both remedy and dose were right and a true cure is in progress. But if we find superficial symptoms disappearing and vital organs show-

ing signs of advancing disease, we know we
have failed.[12]

When cure is in progress, changes occur first at the innermost level.

> The amelioration is apt to show itself in the
> mental state first; the mind becomes more tran-
> quil and the suffering is more easily borne, al-
> though its intensity may as yet not be lessened
> . . . All other ways are irregular and open to the
> suspicion of being mere palliations calculated
> to destroy the natural symmetry of the manifes-
> tations, hence to complicate and render the dis-
> ease intractable.[13]

As we can see, there is a lot to watch and wait for in
the second, third, and fourth prescriptions. Homoeopathic treatment gradually unravels the case going back
to the beginnings of illness, eliminating symptoms along
the way in the reverse order of their appearance, until
finally real, lasting health is achieved.

How Do We Know the Remedy Has Failed to Act?

Just as important as observing remedy action is observing that a remedy has not acted. Again, a consistent
approach is needed, asking: How do I know the remedy
has not acted? Why didn't the remedy act? Generally
speaking, if the remedy and dose are correctly selected,
after a reasonable length of time, depending on the
acute or chronic nature of the case, we expect changes,
reaction, and results to occur.

> Of course, if a prescription is not related to the case, if it is a prescription that effects no changes, it does not take long to see what to do; much patient waiting for a foolish prescription is but loss of time.[14]

If no changes occur we may determine the remedy hasn't acted. We must now determine *why* it didn't act. Typically, failure of remedy action is due to: (1) an error in selection of the first remedy; (2) selection of the wrong potency; (3) a weakened vital force due to long-term suppression or deep, advanced pathology; or (4) obstacles to cure including maintaining causes and miasmatic barriers. In the event the vital force has been seriously weakened and is unable to respond to the stimulation of the remedy; this is commonly called "lack of reaction."

If, in carefully reviewing the symptom record and reconsidering the patient's state of susceptibility, we find the remedy was rightly chosen according to the totality of symptom image, before deserting the first remedy try a higher, lower, or LM potency.

> It is the practice for some to go lower if a high potency has failed. This method has but few recorded successes but should not be ignored.[15]

How Rapidly Do Remedies Act?

The following factors determine rapidity of action in acute cases: the nature of the ailment; the state in which the patient presents for treatment—i.e., the state of the vital force, susceptibility, and the uppermost miasm; and the accuracy of the prescription.

Depending on the curable or incurable* nature of the ailment and the degree to which the disease has penetrated the organism, after the initial slight, temporary intensification and exteriorization of the characteristic symptoms in chronic conditions, the remedy action usually begins within hours or a few days, and takes several weeks, months, or years before it is complete. In acute states, of course, the response is almost immediate. Gradually, under homoeopathic treatment, individuals are made whole once more.

What Are the Major Action Options for Consideration?

After the administration of the homoeopathically selected remedy, one of two events occurs: the state of the illness is changed or it remains the same. Predicting the outcome of treatment comes through experience. Accurate prognosis occurs after the medicine has been administered. Accurate analysis of information received from the patient after the medicine has been administered leads to an accurate prognosis, and guides the practitioner directly to the next step in treatment and the patient to the next phase of cure. After conducting the follow-up examination and carefully evaluating the patient's response to the remedy, there are a number of possible actions to consider. Again, we need to consistently and thoughtfully review these options before se-

---

* Curable and incurable conditions are defined in Chapter 5.

lecting the appropriate course of action. The main action options at the second prescription stage rely on our ability to watch and wait for directional signals from the vital force and our understanding of the Direction of Cure. We will decide whether or not a medicine is required. If so, we can:

• Repeat the same remedy in the same potency.

• Repeat the same remedy in a *different* potency.

• Select a different remedy.

• Select an acute remedy or a chronic remedy.

• Select the acute remedy of the chronic, constitutional remedy.

• Select a related or complementary remedy.

We must be able to provide a clearly reasoned basis for each action we take at each stage of treatment, recorded concisely in our patient record. Each of the possible actions will be discussed in the following chapter illustrated by typical remedy action scenarios.

CHAPTER 3

1. Close, *The Genius of Homoeopathy*, Chapter 13, pg. 205.
2. Kent, *Minor Writings*, pg. 238.
3. Hahnemann, *Organon*, 6th ed. (Boericke trans.), ¶33.
4. Hahnemann, *The Chronic Diseases*, Volume 1, Preface to the Fourth Volume, pg. 18.
5. Hahnemann, *Organon*, 6th ed. (Boericke trans.), ¶62.
6. Close, *The Genius of Homoeopathy*, Chapter 13, pg. 206.

7. Kent, *Lectures on Homoeopathic Philosophy,*
   Lecture 35, pg. 224.
8. Kent, *Lectures on Homoeopathic Philosophy,*
   Lecture 35, pg. 226.
9. Kent, *Lectures on Homoeopathic Philosophy,*
   Lecture 35, pg. 228.
10. Kent, *Lectures on Homoeopathic Philosophy,*
    Lecture 35, pg. 226.
11. Close, *The Genius of Homoeopathy,* Chapter 13,
    pg. 208.
12. Close, *The Genius of Homoeopathy,* Chapter 13,
    pg. 207, 208.
13. Boger, *Boenninghausen's Characteristics, Materia
    Medica, and Repertory,* Preface, pg. 10.
14. Kent, *Lectures on Homoeopathic Philosophy,* Lecture
    35, pg. 224.
15. Kent, *Minor Writings,* pg. 237.

CHAPTER 4

Crossroads To Cure

BEFORE DECIDING TO MAKE another prescription, we have examined the patient and determined if the remedy has acted. Now we must detect whether the remedy has acted deeply or superficially, totally or partially.

> What is more beautiful to look upon than the bud during its hourly changes to the rose in its bloom? This evolution has so often come to my mind when patiently awaiting the return of symptoms after the first prescription has exhausted its curative power. The return symptom-image unfolds the knowledge by which we know whether the first prescription was the specific or the palliative, i.e., we may know whether the remedy was deep enough to cure all the deranged vital wrong or simply a superficially acting remedy, capable of only temporary effect.[1]

This chapter evaluates a range of typical remedy actions and patient responses, and suggests appropriate practitioner actions.

Due to the unique nature of each individual's fundamental miasm and current state of susceptibility, we must expect a wide range of responses. To simplify and clarify a potentially confusing situation, we may divide the responses into three main categories: aggravation, amelioration, and alteration of disease symptom complex. Due to everyone's unique state of *individuality* and degree of *susceptibility,* inevitably there will be various subcategories and combinations of these three major categories. Applying the Law of Similars to match the wide range of possible responses, there is a similarly wide range of possible courses of action. It is therefore unlikely that a definitive, exhaustive list of patient response possibilities can be created.

However, we have to start somewhere and the following responses are those most commonly found. This chapter draws upon the writings of Hahnemann, Boger, Close, Harvey Farrington, Kent, Roberts, and Wright-Hubbard.

First, desirable, curative responses are described, followed by undesirable responses. Finally, questionable responses that require further case evaluation are discussed. Possible remedy actions are presented using "scenarios," which describe the individual's response, evaluation of the response, and suggested practitioner action. (As stated earlier, case management of LM potencies requires slightly different assessment criteria and practitioner action, which are discussed in Chapter 5.) What follows relates primarily to centesimal dosage.

Curative Responses to Homoeopathic Medicines

Experience teaches that whenever the quite correctly and fittingly chosen remedy is administered and operates within the sphere corresponding to its action, hence [it] excites the necessary reaction, the overthrow of the disease is naturally to be expected.[2]

Ideally the individual and his symptoms improve. We give the remedy; an initial reaction, perhaps a barely perceptible homoeopathic aggravation, ensues, followed by relief, and the person feels distinctly better. Curative change comes about. Signs and symptoms of the disturbance begin to change in an orderly way according to the Direction of Cure. Waste products are thrown off from within to without. Abscesses or suppurations appear on the surface or in glands, but not in vital organs. There is a discharge of some kind, i.e., nasal, vaginal, urethral, or an exteriorization of the disorder through a skin eruption.

People respond to a correctly chosen remedy in a variety of ways. There may or may not be an initial excitation of the original, presenting characteristic symptoms. There may be a period of turmoil as the vital force exteriorizes the disturbance and the symptom picture changes. We may feel better immediately or after a delay.

Each person, like each medicine, is unique. However, there are certain patterns of responses to expect, and similar responses have been loosely grouped together. These bear careful reading. Scenarios that may seem the same are subtly different and need to be separately considered.

Remember, the more closely your selected remedy and potency resemble the symptom image totality, (i.e., the simillimum), the more rapid and gentle the patient's response is likely to be. The scenario "Recovery Without Aggravation" illustrates this ideal curative response for which we all strive.

1. *Action and Turmoil*

After the first homoeopathic prescription, the patient reports experiencing an initial intensification of the presenting symptoms, then everything calms down and she feels much better in every way. She has a few small symptoms that aren't bothering her too much.

EVALUATION—It is a good prescription. The striking features, the characteristic, peculiar original symptoms of the patient that guided us to the remedy have been removed, and only trivial, tolerable symptoms remain. The remedy has brought relief to the patient.

ACTION—WAIT. Do not prescribe on the remaining trivial symptoms. WAIT, long enough for a return of original (presenting) symptoms before prescribing. Too early repetition of the medicine or continually giving the same medicine and ignoring Hahnemann's rule of slightly altering the potency of each dose, risks interference with the curative action of the medicine and prevents the possibility of making a good second prescription. WAIT and give the vital force the opportunity to call for a second prescription through the return of original symptoms.

If you repeat too soon, the patient's guiding symptoms become intermingled with the drug symptoms (symptoms caused by the remedy). This unfortunate situation incurs the exact opposite of our intention, unnecessary patient suffering, and it requires great skill in sorting out the ensuing muddle.

2. Action, Then Standstill

After the remedy there was an initial reaction to the remedy in which the original presenting symptoms intensified temporarily. The turmoil gradually subsides until the patient has no symptoms and says, "I don't feel ill exactly, and yet I don't feel well either, but I can't really say why or how."

EVALUATION—There is doubt as to whether the remedy is still acting or has ceased to act. The presenting symptoms appear to have lessened in their intensity and the patient has improved to some degree, but nothing is happening now. The patient is most likely in the "standstill phase," but if there are few or no clear symptoms, there is no clear guide to the next action or prescription.

It is rarely the case that a new prescription becomes necessary when the case merely comes to a standstill. The first prescription has been made and the symptoms commence to change in an orderly way; they change and interchange and new symptoms come up, but finally the symptoms go back to their original state, not marked enough to be of any importance, without any special suffering to the patient, and the patient has arrived at a state of standstill. The patient says, "I have no symptoms, yet I am not improving; I seem to have come to a standstill position." He says this as to himself, not as to the symptoms.[3]

ACTION—WAIT.

At this point without signs or symptoms, Kent says there is nothing to tell us what to do, so we must do nothing.[4]

In the meantime, in order to accurately assess the situation, examine the patient carefully. You may find, after all, that her symptoms have changed in an orderly way, and the original symptoms have receded to a state where the patient is not bothered by them. The worst symptoms are evidently better, which is why the patient reports few or no symptoms. The patient has, in fact, improved.

ACTION—WAIT.

> It is the duty of the physician then to wait, and wait a long time . . . A new prescription cannot be entertained, because there is no guide to it . . . Wait a long time when patients come to a standstill.[5]

Do not prescribe; give the patient perfect rest from further prescriptions or you will irrevocably spoil the case.

> The patient will get along just as well without any medicine, and get along better without that medicine that helped him than with it. In curable cases, whose prospects are good, he will go along for a long time, and become very much relieved of his symptoms.[6]

Whenever in doubt, do not prescribe. Wait for a clear image to emerge; wait for the vital force to direct you. Wait maybe days, weeks, months. Good timing in prescribing is crucial. While you wait for something to happen, touch base with the patient at regular intervals to ascertain, through the return of original symptoms, when the remedy ceases to act.

We must not impose our schedule of progress on the patient. Individual timetables of response are so varied as to be impossible to predict. We should resist the temptation to prescribe because of some theoretical formula such as "a certain potency acts in a certain amount of time." Individuality of the vital force, susceptibility, miasms, and remedy action reign supreme.

> The finest curative action I ever observed has begun sixty days after the administration of the single dose.[7]

> In such states we should wait until we are quite sure the remedy has ceased to act. There are remedies that have a "do nothing" stage in their unfolding, and we must be sure, before repeating the remedy, that the first prescription has entirely run out its cycle. If we found a "do nothing" stage, it may be part of the remedy cycle; if so the remedy is still acting and to repeat the remedy at this time could do no good and might do harm. In other words, this "do nothing" stage is an expression of the pathogenesis of the remedy manifesting itself in the curative process, and by a little more patient

waiting the patient will be ready for the next prescription. In these "do nothing" states no other remedy can fill in, because there are no strong indications for another remedy and the symptomatology has not altered to any marked degree except by lessening in intensity, and since there has been little change and no marked new symptoms have arisen, we have no guides for another remedy.[8]

In the materia medicas, check for possible "do nothing" stages. For example, Sepia is a remedy renowned for having "quiet" times. In our daily haste and eagerness for rapid cure, if we mistake these lulls in activity for *inactivity* and prescribe before the remedy has exhausted itself, even if we give the same remedy, we risk confusing the case and spoiling the patient's chances of cure.

I know it's difficult for some to confidently trust in an intangible dynamic spirit-like Life Force, but for homoeopathy to be successful it is essential to recognize and acknowledge that in sickness and in health, the life force alone is in control. Observing and listening to the vital force through its expression of symptoms is our only reliable guide along the road to cure. If the remedy is repeated too soon, *before the action of the first remedy is exhausted,* we risk breaking the cycle of cure and inadvertently causing a dangerous intermingling of *drug* symptoms with the *patient's* symptoms, with the tragic consequence the original, once clear image will now be seriously, even irrevocably obscured and muddled. To avoid interrupting the delicate curative cycle, we must constantly resist the urge to prescribe too early. The remedy must always be allowed to act to its fullest extent.

Whenever considering prescribing, be alert to the fact that perfect timing is the goal; be sure the window of susceptibility to the medicine is open. Awaiting the optimum moment to prescribe is a very critical time. Being too quick on the draw, careless, or ineffective in monitoring the case, we may easily miss that optimum prescription opportunity. To avoid bad timing, check the patient's state every few days. Continue to wait while the overall well-being of the patient remains steady or increases. If you determine the remedy has really come to a *standstill,* wait some more for the presenting symptoms to return before prescribing again.

In uncertain situations where there are no marked new symptoms and the symptoms have not altered to any marked degree except by lessening in intensity, there is no guide to another remedy. Waiting for the return of the original symptoms is all there is to do.

3. Amelioration, Then Return of Presenting Symptoms

After the remedy, the patient says, "I was much better, but now I'm worse again."

EVALUATION—The first remedy was correct and acted. The patient reports a brief amelioration, then the reappearance of the original, presenting, characteristic symptoms that were experienced before remedy administration. The case is curable. However, although the first prescription helped for a while, it didn't hold the patient through to complete cure. The presenting symptoms have returned, therefore the vital force is calling for more medicine.

ACTION—Before making the next prescription, have the patient check in regularly to make sure the curative action of the remedy is completely exhausted. WAIT and make sure the symptoms are not coming and going. The original complaints must come back to stay before the next prescription is made. If the symptoms return *to stay,* because the first prescription acted curatively, then we repeat the previous remedy.

> When the symptom picture/image returns unaltered, except for the absence of one or more symptoms, the first remedy should never be changed until ascending potencies have exhausted their powers.[9]

> Wait for the curative impulse to entirely subside and the reappearance, one by one, of original characteristic symptoms, falling into place to arrange before the intelligent physician an image of the disease for the purpose of cure.[10]

When improvement ceases or old symptoms reappear and remain without change, it is time to repeat the dose.

> . . . The interval between doses stand[s] next in importance only to the selection of the right remedy.[11]

The rule is: never change the remedy so long as the patient improves after administration of the medicine. If the patient feels improved, continue that remedy at appropriate intervals. In this way we encourage the curative power forward. Go up through the potencies of your chosen scale, when indicated by the patient's vital force, until you give a higher potency without effect. If you reach the end of the scale and the same remedy is still indicated, go back to your starting potency and begin ascending the scale again. Repeating the ascending scale works because the vital force, less burdened by symptoms, is now more open and susceptible at a deeper level to the potentized homoeopathic medicine the second time round. Through continuous homoeopathic treatment, the patient's state of health has been taken to a different level and the remedy seems to take a deeper hold on the organism.

4. *Characteristic Symptoms Return but Patient Feels Well*

After the remedy the patient reports the existing symptoms disappeared briefly and then returned, but they are not bothered by them to any great degree and in themselves they feel very good.

EVALUATION—Brief amelioration followed by reappearance of the original, characteristic symptoms that the patient experienced before but less intense and disturbing the patient to a lesser degree, indicates a good prescription and the remedy is still acting.

ACTION—WAIT. Avoid too early repetition and let the remedy continue to complete its curative action. Wait and watch carefully for the characteristic symptoms to intensify once again and for the patient's sense of well-being and vitality to begin to decline before making the second prescription. Have the patient check in regularly for a brief progress report, so as not to miss the optimum prescription time.

5. Characteristic Symptoms Come and Go

The patient returns and reports: "I feel pretty good myself, except the herpes I had before keeps coming back from time to time. Anyway, even that is better, it just doesn't seem to be quite as bad as it was before the medicine. Maybe it lasts a day or an hour or less. My old attacks lasted weeks."

EVALUATION—The symptoms reappear from time to time. The remedy has acted and is acting. There is a coming and going of characteristic symptoms because the reordering process of the vital force induces turmoil. We are witnessing a return of the original, presenting symptoms, less strong or marked than previously, but the same symptoms. Each time the herpes comes back it is less severe. The symptom is growing weaker and the patient is improving.

According to Hahnemann, the remedy is acting well and usefully. These are homoeopathic aggravations of the original ailments. Before a chronic miasm so deeply enrooted and, as it were, parasitically interwoven with our life force can be eradicated and health restored, consider the great changes which must be effected by the medicine in the many, variously composite and incredibly delicate parts of our living organism. It is natural that during the long-continued action of a dose of medicine, selected homoeopathically, assaults on the organism may be made by the miasm in undulating fluctuations at various times during this long-continued disease. These homoeopathic excitations do not hinder; they advance cure. If the dose is a moderate one, these assaults will take place more and more rarely—gradually they will disappear naturally.[12]

ACTION—WAIT. Delay as long as practicable before repeating the medicine. Cure cannot be accomplished more quickly and surely than by allowing the suitable remedy to continue its action, so long as the improvement continues, even if this should be several or many days. Only when the original, presenting symptoms, which had been eradicated or very much diminished, are renewed and commence to rise again for a few days or again be perceptibly experienced, has the time surely come when another dose of the medicine should be given.[13]

Hahnemann gives us the example of a case in which Sepia was indicated for a peculiar headache that appeared in repeated attacks. After the medicine was given, the ailment was diminished both as to intensity and duration, and the pauses between attacks greatly lengthened. When the attacks reappeared the dose was repeated, which caused them to cease for 100 days, after which the headache reappeared again to some degree. This necessitated another dose, after which no other attack took place for seven years, while the health was also otherwise perfect.[14]

In his discussion of the action of antipsoric remedies in Volume I of *The Chronic Diseases*, Hahnemann gives us much succinct guidance on how long to wait after the first dose of a remedy is given before prescribing. This wisdom is as important to homoeopaths today as it was when Hahnemann first wrote it. I have paraphrased his words in the following paragraphs.

As a rule in chronic disease, the more tedious (complex) the diseases are, the longer the medicines continue their action. In acute diseases, medicines act only a short time—the more acute the disease, the shorter the action. In chronic diseases, so long as they perceptibly continue to improve the diseased state of the patient, even though gradually, the physician must allow all antipsoric remedies to act thirty, forty, or even fifty and more days *by themselves*. They must not be disturbed and checked by any new remedy.

If appropriately selected medicines are *not* allowed to act their full time when they are acting well, the whole treatment will amount to nothing. If another remedy is administered too early, before the present remedy ceases to act, or a new dose of the same remedy is given, the good effect of the preceding remedy will be lost and cannot be replaced because its complete action has been interrupted.

Hahnemann says it is a fundamental rule in treatment of chronic diseases to let the action of the remedy come to an undisturbed conclusion, so long as it visibly advances the cure and while improvement still perceptibly progresses. This method forbids any new prescription—any interruption by another medicine—and also forbids the immediate repetition of the same remedy.

He tells us that there has been much abuse of this immediate repetition of doses of the same medicine because young (novice) homoeopaths, thinking to heal more quickly, think it more convenient to repeat a medicine which in the beginning had been found to be homoeopathically suitable. They tend to do this without reexamining the case and even repeat it *frequently*. Hahnemann says the practice of giving the patient several doses of the same medicine to take with him so that he may dose himself at certain intervals, without considering the possibility this repetition may affect him injuriously, seems to show a negligent empiricism and is unworthy of a homoeopathic physician. Hahnemann instructs us not to allow a new dose of a medicine to be taken or given without convincing ourselves in every case beforehand as to its *usefulness*.

Sometimes the dose of a well-selected, beneficial remedy has made some beginning toward improvement, but its action ceases too quickly—its power is too soon exhausted—and the cure does not proceed any further. This is rare in chronic diseases, but is frequently the case in acute diseases, as well as in chronic diseases that rise into any acute state: the acute of a chronic state. After fourteen, ten, seven, and even fewer days, when the peculiar symptoms of the acute disease visibly cease to diminish, and the improvement has clearly come to a stop, (so long as there is no disturbance of the mind and no appearance of any new, troublesome symptoms), it is useful to give a dose of the same medicine in a similarly small amount, but most safely in a different degree of dynamic potency.[15] When the remedy is thus modified, the vital force of the patient will allow itself more easily to be further affected by the same medicine and complete its expected cure.[16]

6. *The Symptoms Get Worse yet the Patient Feels Better*

   After the remedy, the patient reports, "My hot sweats are worse, but I feel great!" There's great improvement in the general sense of well-being, yet the presenting characteristic symptoms of the patient are intensified and become more marked.

   EVALUATION—This is a good sign the remedy is acting curatively. If the patient feels well in herself, yet the characteristic individualizing symptoms are briefly, slightly worse, this indicates the patient is experiencing the so-called "homoeopathic aggravation," more accurately described by Hahnemann as the "initial excitation response" to the remedy action.[17] Strangely, and counter to our expectations of a curative process, in homoeopathy this excitation response of existing characteristic symptoms is a highly favorable reaction to a well-chosen remedy. In homoeopathy we are treating the *individual* with her symptoms. In this scenario the *patient* feels better. This response is quite different from an aggravation of the pathological symptoms in which the patient also feels worse.

   It's essential to distinguish between the two types of aggravations: (1) an aggravation of the *disease,* in which the patient *and* the pathological symptoms grow worse—a bad sign, and (2) an aggravation of the *characteristic individualizing symptoms* in which the patient is growing better, which results from the intensified centrifugal curative action of the remedy. This type of response is common in acute disorders. If cure is taking place, these symptoms will subside rapidly after remedy administration, and improvement will quickly follow. In chronic cases the aggravation of characteristic symptoms may last several days and then subside.

This slight homoeopathic aggravation during the first hours, is quite in order, and in case of an acute disease, generally serves as an excellent indication that it will yield to the first dose. The drug-disease [the remedy] must naturally be somewhat more intense in order to overcome and extinguish the natural disease; as it is only by superior intensity that one natural disease can extinguish another of similar nature.[18]

The smaller the dose of the homoeopathic remedy, so much the smaller and shorter is the apparent aggravation of the disease during the first hours.[19]

ACTION—WAIT. Leave the patient alone. Let the remedy continue acting, encouraging the vital force to exteriorize the dynamic, inner disturbance through the physical body. To avoid any unnecessary suffering, check the degree of symptom intensity and direction of reappearing symptoms compared to the symptoms in your case taking. If it is a chronic case, have the patient check in with you at least on a weekly basis to ensure that the initial aggravation response abates. Wait for the remedy to cease acting and for the eventual return of the original symptoms before making a further prescription.

In an acute case the aggravation could be very brief or imperceptible, followed by clear improvement of the patient and the symptoms.

7. *Short Aggravation and Rapid Amelioration*

The patient returns and reports: "After the remedy, everything got much worse on all levels for a week. Then gradually, during the last three weeks, the symptoms I originally complained of disappeared. The pain in my neck has gone, but there is some elbow pain, and there is a rash of some kind on my leg. I feel okay overall and really the rash doesn't bother me all that much."

EVALUATION—This indicates a short, vigorous, initial response followed by a rapid amelioration. Direction of Cure is clear. This is a good sign and much desired.

> Improvement will be marked, the reaction of the economy is vigorous, and there is no tendency to any structural change in the vital organs. Any structural changes that may be present will be found on the surface in organs that are not vital; abscesses will form and often glands that can be done without will suppurate in regions that are not important to the life of the patient. Such organic changes are surface changes, and are not like the changes that take place in the liver, in the kidneys, in the heart, and in the brain: an aggravation quick, short, and strong is one that is to be wished for and is followed by quick improvement.[20]

ACTION—WAIT. Do not interfere with the curative response. Wait and watch for the original symptoms to return.

8. *Recovery Without Aggravation*

The patient returns and reports: "I took the medicine and all my troubles disappeared. I feel like a million dollars. I didn't even have the twinge you mentioned I might have."

EVALUATION—In functional diseases, or in the beginning of acute organic diseases, accompanied perhaps by severe pain, the administration of the appropriate dose of the indicated remedy may be followed by rapid disappearance of symptoms without any aggravation. This is a cure of the most satisfactory kind, pleasing alike to physician and patient. Remedy and potency were both exactly right.[21]

This is an ideal response to the remedy. The remedy is acting. The initial response was imperceptible, yet the patient recovers steadily. The remedy and potency were precisely correct. According to Roberts and Kent, this scenario illustrates that the chronic disease belongs to the function of the nerves rather than threatened tissue changes. Although patients may suffer severely in these states before treatment, they are often cured without the commonly observed initial short-lived intensification of symptoms following administration of the medicine. In this situation, providing the original symptoms *do not return* and the patient returns to health in an orderly way and continues to feel better in herself on all levels, we are observing the "No Aggravation, with Recovery of the Patient" response.

ACTION—Celebrate! Then WAIT maybe a few weeks or months. WAIT actively for that window of opportunity to open before making another prescription at precisely the optimum moment. Waiting actively means set up regular, short-interval patient progress reports. Wait for the vital force to call for help to finish the cure. Wait until the patient's energy dips, and there is a reappearance of the original symptoms perhaps returning a little changed from the former state. Then, because the first prescription had a beneficial effect and must be permitted to continue its work to the fullest extent, the only course of action is repetition of the first prescription in remedy and potency.

The Golden Rule is *never, ever change a remedy without a very good reason.* Put simply, in this instance you cannot give another remedy because, through the positive patient response, it has demonstrated itself to be the patient's correct remedy. It should not be changed so long as the curative action can be maintained. Remember, if the patient has improved continuously according to the Law of Direction of Cure, even if the symptoms have changed, *do not change the remedy,* even though it would be impossible for you, at this time, to select that first remedy again from the present symptoms observed. Hold on fast to that first medicine so long as you secure improvement and good from it. As long as the patient improves the first remedy can be repeated at the appropriate intervals, ascending through the whole range of potencies with improvement from each potency before you pass to the next one. As stated in the fifth scenario, when you have reached the end of a particular potency scale, go back to the beginning, and ascend the same potency scale again, starting with the potency you first administered. The medicine will work effectively due to the patient's improved state of health, vital force, susceptibility, and quieted miasm.

9. Correct Direction of Response

The patient returns saying, "My knee is more painful; I have pimples, but I'm sleeping better, and I feel much less irritable than before."

EVALUATION—Some symptoms are better and some are worse. The remedy is correct and is acting. The correct, curative direction, innermost to outermost, is in progress. The sleep and irritability on the mental plane are better, and the knee and pimples on the physical plane are worse. The innermost disturbance is exteriorizing through the outermost extremities. Cure is proceeding in an orderly manner from within to without, and the patient is improving.

ACTION—WAIT. Carefully assess the shift in location and direction of the symptoms, and educate the patient about the principle of Direction of Cure. Wait. *Never* risk interrupting the curative process by prescribing *too early.* Remember, in homoeopathy, more of the same is not always better. Too early repetition does not maintain medicine momentum or help the vital force. In fact, it has the exact opposite effect of deraling or overwhelming the vital force and preventing curative progress.

It is an error to think of a medicine when a symptom–image is changing. The physician must wait for permanency or firmness in the

relations of the image before making a prescription. Some say, "I must give the patient
medicine or he will go and see someone else." I
have only to say that it were better had all sick
folks gone somewhere else, for these doctors
seldom cure but often complicate the sickness
[by prescribing too early].[22]

10. Return of Old Symptoms

Some days after the medicine, the patient reports
feeling a moderate ailment, headache, or else a sore
throat, diarrhea, or pain of some kind.

EVALUATION—A well-chosen medicine is acting. If the
symptoms have occurred, if not in the last few weeks, at
least now and then some weeks or months before this
recent occurrence (before the remedy was taken), then
these headache, sore throat, diarrhea, or pain symptoms
are through the medicine, merely a homoeopathic excitation of some symptom common to this disease symptom image, a homoeopathic excitation of something
which had perhaps been more frequently troublesome
to the patient in the past. In other words, the patient is
experiencing a return of old symptoms. The appearance
of these symptoms is a sign that this medicine acts
deeply into the very essence of the disease, and that it
will, consequently, be effective in the future.[23]

ACTION—Don't think appearance of these moderate
symptoms means you must at once give the patient
some other medicine.

No! The homoeopathic . . . medicine having been chosen as well as possible to suit the morbid symptoms, and given in the appropriate potency and in the proper dose, the physician should *as a rule* allow it to finish its action without disturbing it by an intervening remedy.[24]

11. Disappearance of Characteristic Symptoms

After the remedy the patient reports, "Apart from a few trivial symptoms, all my major problems I came for have improved or disappeared."

EVALUATION—This is a good sign of recovery beginning. The patient is experiencing curative changes in the original, guiding symptomatology. Complaints upon which we based the prescription are almost erased.

ACTION—WAIT! The first prescription was correct. The delicate cycle of cure must be left to continue uninterrupted before making a new prescription. In this situation, the homoeopath's superior powers of observation are triggered. Oftentimes symptoms may not return as strongly as they appeared before the first prescription. They may not be as obvious to us as they were before. While the patient experiences these trivial symptoms, wait and watch carefully for the return of definite, strong presenting symptoms to become apparent to the patient before giving more medicine.

The answer to the key question of how long we should wait before making the next prescription varies between different individuals depending on their state and circumstances and the action of different remedies within the individual. Accordingly we may wait a few weeks or months.

Beware! We can't predict anything. Don't be fooled into acting before the vital force is ready to proceed. In order to keep on top of the situation and grasp the optimum moment to make the next prescription, short interval check-in is essential—ask the patient to check with you every week to ten days. Active watching and waiting is required to avoid missing the moment the remedy ceases to act.

> Let the remedy be allowed to complete its work
> to its fullest extent before making the second
> prescription.[25]

12. *Only Local Symptoms Remain*

The patient returns and reports: "It's been a while now and overall I feel good. Everything bit by bit has improved, but I still have this patch of really irritating eczema on my stomach which won't go away, and the pains in my joints are still there on and off."

EVALUATION—The remedy has been given plenty of time to act, without interference; characteristic symptoms are mostly eliminated, but a few, local exterior symptoms, e.g., symptoms on the physical plane involving the skin and extremities, remain. The central disturbance has shifted to the outermost. The local symptoms are on the physical plane, not the mental plane. The case has not quite achieved complete curative status. It needs a little more help to finish the job.

ACTION—Search for a more similar remedy to complete the cure. Rather than prescribing a well-proven remedy with a wide spectrum of operation, a polychrest, perhaps seek out a remedy that is less well proven and therefore less represented in the repertory. In this search for a better indicated remedy, select a rubric in the repertory that more closely reflects the persisting local symptoms. For example, if the patient is "sick from noise," choose the rubric *Stomach, nausea, noise from,*[26] rather than *Mind, sensitive, noise to.* Taking the more precise localized symptom rubric along with the remaining totality of the case, you'll find the better selected remedy needed to complete cure.

Now that we understand simple patient responses to remedy actions, let's get down to the nitty-gritty, more challenging aspect of homoeopathy, the management of complicated situations.

Problem Responses to Homoeopathic Medicines

Acknowledging the fact that, for a variety of reasons, unfavorable responses are bound to occur, reduces practitioner anxiety resulting in clearer focus on how to manage these complications effectively and proceed confidently, even in the most challenging circumstances. The following section explores questionable, problematic responses to remedies and offers suggestions as to how they may be effectively interpreted and resolved. Described below are several unfavorable responses that may indicate a potentially curable case that requires a more creative approach to symptom evaluation and case analysis *or* an incurable state needing palliation.

Having introduced the terms *incurable* and *curable,*
let's define and clarify them from the homoeopathic
perspective. In the *Organon,* Hahnemann says all *curable* diseases make themselves known to the intelligent
physician in signs and symptoms.[27] Unlike in mainstream medical thought, in homoeopathy symptoms
such as pain, vomiting, diarrhea, sweating, fever, lack of
appetite, and all manner of other discomforts experienced by the individual in a particular state of disorder
are the physician's friend rather than enemy. Of course,
symptoms and discomfort signal the organism's indi-
vidualistic struggle to regain balance, but it is through
the unique symptom patterns that the vital force com-
municates its distress to the intelligent, perceiving homoeopath. The displayed signs and symptoms are vi-
tally important. They signal not only the approximate
location of disorder/imbalance, but also the degree of
individual suffering, the strength of the vital force, and
the extent of its success in battling the enemy within.

Symptoms are therefore essential for cure in homoeopathy. Each individual's unique disorder pattern is
the only infallible guide to the correct remedy. Therefore from a homoeopathic perspective, a case is *curable*
when it displays an individualizing symptom pattern.
The reappearance or disappearance of symptoms also
indicates whether there has been a favorable or unfavorable response to the remedy.

As a crime without clues cannot be solved, a case
without distinctive characteristic symptoms cannot be
cured because they enable homoeopaths to clearly see
the likeness of every disease and, through review of the
symptomatology in the provings data, the homoeopath

sees the likeness of the curative remedy in the symptom pattern. Symptoms reappearing and disappearing also allow us to determine whether there has been a curative or noncurative response to remedies. An *incurable* state is best defined by Kent.

> Incurable results of disease are incurable for two reasons: first, destruction of tissues of the organism. Second, deficient reaction of the vital force, [either through] acquired debility or congenital weakness.[28]

In other words the degree to which an individual is incurable depends on the degree of destruction wrought by the disturbance from within. Unfortunately, in organic disorders of the body, signs and symptoms of the condition decrease in proportion as the pathology advances. This is evidenced by the lack of individualizing symptom expression experienced among patients suffering advanced malignant tumors. Often some serious disorders may not manifest discomfort at any level, and the true severity of the disturbance remains undiscovered until a regular physical examination reveals the existence of some advanced pathology. From the homoeopathic perspective, this lack of symptom expression is due to the enfeebled state of the vital force, which is too weak to fight unaided. It is too weak to attempt to exteriorize the disturbance and too weak to produce the distress signals necessary for cure through homoeopathy. Usually the organism produces symptoms at some level, which can be recognized by the homoeopath.

To summarize: whether the physician fails to obtain or observe the symptoms, whether there are few or no symptoms, or whether the patient conceals the symptoms, without symptoms we have lost our only guides to possible cure, and the state may consequently be incurable. However, even if the change of state is perceived to be incurable, there is always a potential for homoeopathic treatment to reduce suffering and restore a degree of equilibrium and improve the individual's quality of remaining life even though eventually death is unavoidable.

Examples of common problematic responses to remedy actions are provided below in the context of "scenarios" accompanied by evaluations and suggested actions.

1. Amelioration of Too Short Duration

In his sixth observation, documented in the *Lectures on Homoeopathic Philosophy*, Kent describes a situation arising in a chronic case when a deep-acting remedy has been given in a higher centesimal dose (Sulphur CM). The patient returns at the end of the first, second, and third weeks and says he has done well and has been improving all the time from the Sulphur CM. At the end of the fourth week the patient returns and says, "I've been running down."

EVALUATION—Too short amelioration duration. Be suspicious in curable cases. According to Kent's experience, the higher and highest potencies act a long time because the remedy acts at once and establishes a condition of order upon the patient. This order continues for a considerable length of time, sometimes several months. In curable cases where prospects are good, patients go along for a long time and become very much relieved of their symptoms without needing another medicine. Therefore, to have a *correctly chosen medicine* act only a few weeks in a chronic case, when it ought to act for longer, makes us suspicious. Either the remedy was only partially similar, something occurred to disrupt its action, the dose was wrong, or the case is in fact for some reason *incurable*.

ACTION—Examine the patient carefully to discover which of the above possibilities applies. If examination reveals the first prescription covered only part of the case, the first remedy was a partial prescription. Restudy the case and select a more appropriate remedy and potency based on the new information gleaned and the totality of symptom image.

If patient examination reveals that the remedy was correctly chosen and the patient has done nothing to intentionally or unintentionally disrupt the action of the medicine, (for example, there has been no excessive alcohol or drugs, toxic exposure, shock, trauma, or excessive stress) then, Kent tells us, it is likely that structural changes are going on within and organs have been destroyed, are being destroyed, or are in a very precarious condition.[29]

To throw more light on the case and grasp a clearer image of what's happening, obtain as much information as possible about the patient's state of imbalance. As well as meticulous homoeopathic examination of the patient to elicit more characteristic symptoms, expand your information base and advise the patient to take advantage of the diagnostic techniques offered by allopaths and a complete physical investigation. When the patient returns with the results, evaluate him. Utilizing the extra information to reduce discomfort, select a more appropriate remedy and dosage and diligently monitor patient progress, keeping alert for degrees of improvement or decline.

Amelioration of too short duration may also occur in acute cases. Kent gives the example of a dose of medicine given in a severe case of meningitis which may remove all the symptoms for an hour, after which the medicine has to be repeated. After the next dose the patient improves for half an hour and another dose is necessary. We find that the amelioration has reduced from an hour to thirty minutes. As Kent puts it, "you may make up your mind, then, that patient is in a desperate condition."[30]

ACTION—In this situation, carefully and quickly re-study the case for information that will lead you to a better selection of remedy or dose and monitor the patient closely for signs of improvement.

We learn more about managing similar situations from Elizabeth Wright-Hubbard. She tells of a Silica case, which was markedly better for a week or ten days but would then slip back; a change of potency didn't hold the patient longer either.

Her evaluation was that the remedy was only similar enough to palliate symptoms for a little while but not similar enough to affect the innermost, underlying predispositions of the individual, and the constitutional, miasmatic state.[31]

Wright-Hubbard's suggested approach is to interrupt the action of the first remedy by finding another one to take hold of the case. To do this, retake the case and select a more similar, deeper acting, miasmatic remedy that more closely reflects the totality of the disease symptom image, including the prevailing miasmatic predispositions.

In the Silica case described above, Wright-Hubbard gave the closely related and well-indicated nosode, Tuberculinum, a very deep-acting miasmatic remedy, which took hold of the curative process. After that, other remedies given according to the state/image presented were effective.[32]

2. *Prolonged Homoeopathic Aggravation with Slowly Developing Amelioration*

An individual presents with symptoms he has had for a good many years. A well-indicated remedy is prescribed in a very high potency. The presenting symptoms intensify and the patient feels moderately better in himself but not wonderful. The aggravation of presenting symptoms lasts for several weeks and then slow but sure improvement begins on all levels.

EVALUATION—There is minimal vitality to react to the remedy. The chronic state had the beginnings of marked tissue changes, but they had not progressed too far. The patient presented in the nick of time before advanced destructive changes in the vital organs had progressed too far. The prolonged aggravation indicates the potency was too high for such a weakened vital force. It was almost completely overwhelmed.

ACTION—When you observe a prolonged homoeo-pathic aggravation, monitor the case carefully and be prepared to antidote the medicine with a better selected one if things look as though they are taking a turn for the worse. If at the end of a few weeks the patient is a little better than when he took the dose, there is some hope that finally the interior symptoms may have an outward manifestation and the patient will go on to recover.

At the appropriate time, when the patient is pre-pared for another dose of medicine, you will see a rep-etition of the same response to the medicine, which will tell you that this individual was on the borderland of curability. In such cases, Kent tells us:

> It is always well in doubtful cases to go to the lower potencies (30c–200c), and in this way cautiously be prepared to interrupt the action of medicine if the case takes the wrong direc-tion.[33]

3. Prolonged Aggravation, Then Decline

After taking the remedy, a patient returns and re-ports the commonly experienced intensification of the presenting symptoms, but lacking the expected accom-panying increased vitality or sense of well-being since taking the medicine. The presenting symptom excita-tion fails to wear off, and the patient's condition pro-gressively declines on mental/emotional, vital, and physical levels.

EVALUATION—The selected remedy was too deep for the state of the vital force. The potency was too high;

cure is doubtful or the case is incurable. Possibly the case was incorrectly assessed at the beginning of treatment, and/or organic pathology was present rather than threatening.

Generally, the initial response to the remedy (homoeopathic aggravation) occurs within minutes in acute conditions and in the first week to ten days in chronic conditions. If there is a prolonged homoeopathic aggravation without any amelioration whatsoever, and the patient progressively declines, the probability is that the remedy has been too late.[34] The patient's vital force has been overwhelmed by the depth and extent of remedy action and subsequent inner turmoil. This response is somewhat similar to the previous scenario and commonly happens in cases of marked pathology where the patient's vital force is nevertheless strong enough to exteriorize a distinctive symptom image.

> Be very sure it truly was an aggravation and then a decline, and not a long aggravation followed by slow improvement that would indicate a serious case, on the borderline of incurability, caught just in time.[35]

> This kind of response is sometimes observed . . . in chronic, deep-seated disease as a result of the overaction of a deeply acting antipsoric or antisyphilitic medicine, given in too high a potency in the beginning of treatment. If the potency is too high its action may be too deep and far-reaching, and the reaction too great for the

weakened vital power to carry on . . . Very high
potencies of the closely similar remedy are mer-
ciless searchers-out of hidden things. They will
sometimes bring to light a veritable avalanche
of symptoms, which overwhelm the weakened
patient. The disease has gone too far for such
radical probing.[36]

ACTION—Take the same action as described in the previous scenario number 2, consider also scenario number
5, and remember:

The case must be handled with extreme care
as it is seldom that such patients recover per-
fectly.[37]

In beginning treatment of suspicious or possibly incurable cases it is better to use medium
potencies [30c, 200c, or LM] . . . and go higher
gradually, if necessary, as treatment progresses
and the patient improves.[38]

4. Severe Aggravation with Organic Pathology

A person's disordered state involves pathology in a
vital organ, and after frequent repetition of a remedy in
low potency the patient reports or the practitioner ob-
serves and perceives severe intensification of the existing symptoms.

EVALUATION—The dose of a correctly chosen, well-
indicated remedy was *incorrectly* given. This unfavorable response is an overreaction by the vital force due to
too much medicine and could be so severe as to com-

promise the life of the patient, especially if she is a child or sensitive person, and if vital organs such as the brain or lungs are the seat of the disturbance. Close describes such an overreaction of the life force in a case of meningitis, where Belladonna 3c or 6c was given too frequently.

> The more accurate the selection of the medicine, the closer it is to the simillimum, the greater must be the care exercised not to injure the patient by prescribing potencies too low and doses too numerous.[39]

At times like these we are reminded that the efficacy of homoeopathy lies in adherence to the Law of Minimum Dose—the least dose necessary to effect cure is the most beneficial dose. Close warns:

> The careless prescriber rarely recognizes such aggravations. When he notices the symptoms he usually attributes them to the natural course of the disease or calls it a "complication."[40]

This situation is most likely to occur among self-prescribers or through the actions of homoeopathic practitioners who lack adequate understanding of the basic principles of practice and the difference between a homoeopathic aggravation and an aggravation of pathology. Consequently, severe responses like this are inappropriately left too long to subside because the ignorant prescriber mistook the situation for a "healing crisis." In fact, these responses require rapid, skillful intervention.

ACTION—*On the first appearance* of such aggravations, medication should be stopped immediately. If the aggravations do not speedily diminish, interrupt the action of the remedy with an antidote if it is known or a better-selected remedy should be administered.[41]

I would go further and say, if necessary, for the patient's sake, to ensure rapid reestablishment of the curative process and to reduce suffering, we should put pride behind us and urgently seek advice from a more experienced colleague.

5. Incorrect Direction of Cure

After the remedy, the patient reports that symptoms that were harmless and painless before have become painful and pronounced, or physical symptoms are better while mental and emotional symptoms are unchanged or worse. For example, occasional flushes of heat and rheumatism of the knee have been replaced by frequent heart palpitations and depression symptoms.

EVALUATION—This is a bad sign. The Direction of Cure is wrong because the pathological symptoms of the disease are growing stronger, and the person feels bad in themselves. The disease has been allowed to progress inwards and upwards, from less to more vital organs, from the extremities to the heart and brain. If the patient's responses to the remedy involve a change in the general symptom image and the general state of the patient is worsening, it might be because: (1) the first prescription was only similar to *a part of* the whole disease symptom image because the remedy was improperly selected, possibly on the basis of one symptom, i.e., rheumatism; or (2) the disease is incurable.

> Knowledge of disease [pathology] may answer this question. If the disease is incurable, the action of the remedy was not expected to do more than change the sufferings into peaceful symptoms.[42]

ACTION—When destructive symptoms in incurable disease intensify, an antidote (a better-selected medicine) must be *urgently* sought and administered to interrupt the action of the preceding dose. In this instance, the first prescription hasn't acted curatively. The next prescription is the antidote remedy, but the real second prescription will be considered only when we have waited for the new sufferings to demand a remedy.[43]

To save the day in these potentially alarming circumstances, the best thing to do is to gather our wits together, resist panic, act quickly, and above all *think* logically and methodically. If the severity of the condition demands it, with a better-selected remedy interrupt the action of remedy or give its known antidote. If the patient is taking the remedy in the LM potency, stop the dosing. (See Chapter 5.) Wait for the symptoms to die down and then wait until the old true image emerges once more. Study the case afresh and when appropriate, administer the new remedy.

Later, after the new remedy, the patient returns saying, "I must be allergic or something to that medicine; my skin is all inflamed," and after close examination there is no reference to the heart or mind symptoms.

You can relax and breathe again because this time round you chose and administered a better remedy than the first prescription, and the symptoms are moving curatively from center to circumference.

It's at tricky moments like this that rigorous thinking and record keeping really pay off. Only with thorough, consistent case analysis methodology can we rapidly unearth the mistake and, through the application of clearly comprehensible principles, easily and rapidly rectify it.

If we haven't detected the central disturbance, we haven't analyzed the case effectively. We haven't logically evaluated the symptom totality. So we are lost, up the creek without a paddle and more importantly, so is the patient! The more complex the situation, the greater the need to scrutinize the case meticulously and adhere to our fundamental principles.

For the patient's sake and with his permission, swallow pride and discuss the case with a more experienced colleague. It can only decrease anxiety, improve your case management skills, and most important of all, rapidly get the patient back on track towards cure. If nothing else, this particular example illustrates the hazards of prescribing remedies symptomatically, one after another, for *all* the changing symptoms in any sickness, simply because they seem similar to the presenting symptoms.

> Too often the remedy has been only similar enough to the superficial symptoms to change the totality and the image comes back altered, therefore resembling another remedy, which

must always be regarded as a misfortune, by which the case is sometimes spoiled, and the hand of the master may fail to correct the wrong done.[44]

6. *No Change in Symptoms*

Several weeks after the first remedy, the patient reports no change in the symptoms. Careful, consistent questioning determines that there has indeed been no change on the mental/emotional, physical general, or physical particular level, and no change in overall well-being.

EVALUATION—The first prescription was ill chosen.

ACTION—Restudy the case. This time, endeavor to elicit facts specifically in relation to the more characteristic, distinguishing features of the case. Carefully, and without prejudice about the patient or towards a particular remedy, study the case more thoroughly. Perhaps there is a new light on the emotions or sensations to which they may have become so accustomed they are unaware of them.

Should renewed efforts confirm that the first remedy is the most similar in its characteristic totality *watch and wait for the return of old symptoms*. But don't leave the patient in limbo, not knowing what's going on. Once again, explain what you are doing and why. Ask the patient to check in regularly with you so you can monitor the return of symptoms, which will tell you when to prescribe a repetition of the first remedy, usually in a slightly altered potency.

7. *Local Physical Symptoms Better but Patient Feels Worse*

The patient says, "Overall I feel worse mentally and emotionally, my energy is down, but some of the irritating skin patches are better."

EVALUATION—This is a bad sign. The outermost is better than the innermost. The patient is going in the opposite Direction of Cure. In the curative response, the *patient* should always feel better even if the symptoms get temporarily, slightly worse. This response may be due to too early repetition of the remedy, too frequent dosing (resulting in homoeopathic symptom suppression), or basing the remedy selection on only part of the whole image totality, thereby giving what is called a partial similar remedy.

ACTION—Restudy the case for errors. Rectify them and interrupt the current remedy by selecting one that more accurately reflects the whole totality of the symptom image.

8. *Overreaction to the Remedy*

The patient is in turmoil, with some or all symptoms worse.

EVALUATION—This is a sign that:

(1) The correct remedy was given in too low a potency, i.e., less dilute, too crude a dose, as in the decimal (x) and lower centesimal potencies (3c–12c), perhaps repeatedly. This has been an excessive dose of the medicine and has established a drug disease.[45]

(2) The remedy is the wrong one.

(3) The patient is oversensitive to the correctly chosen remedy.

(4) The potency has been too high for the state of the vital force, as described in problem scenarios 2 and 3.

ACTION—Remember, whenever there has been an over-reaction, the greater the turmoil, the deeper the tissue change, the more intense or painful the reaction, the more deeply seated the trouble is, the more carefully must we seek the simillimum. At all costs we need to keep our heads in the midst of patient turmoil. Kent advises us to proceed cautiously to a medicine.

> The greatest sufferings may intervene in the change of symptoms during progress of permanent recovery, and if such symptoms are disturbed by a new prescription or palliated by inappropriate medicine, the patient may never be cured.[46]

In the case of evaluation (1), a drug disease will need to be extinguished. Hahnemann deals with this in *Chronic Diseases* where he instructs us to extinguish this injurious, medicinal disease by checking the action of the medicine. Either prescribe its antidote, or if this is not as yet known, give another, antipsoric medicine fitting the patient's state as well as possible. This time, give it in a *very moderate dose*. If this action is not enough to extinguish the medicinal disease, restudy the case and search for still another remedy as homoeopathically suitable as possible.[47]

Interestingly, in the same passage Hahnemann goes on to instruct: Later on, when the stormy assault caused by too large a dose of homoeopathically selected medicine has been assuaged through administration of another, better-selected remedy, the former remedy (which had been hurtful only because of its over-large dose), can be used again. This remedy can be given as soon as it is homoeopathically indicated, and indeed can be used with the greatest success *but only if it is this time given in a far smaller dose and in a much more highly potentized milder quality attenuation.*[48]

ACTION—In evaluation (2), a wrong remedy choice, Hahnemann reassures us: If ever it should happen that the choice of remedy has not been correctly made, the great advantage remains that the incorrectly selected medicine in this smallest dose may be counteracted more easily (than if it's given in too large a dose), with a more suitable medicine. After doing this the cure may be continued without delay.[49] Restudy the case to find the more appropriate remedy.

ACTION—In evaluation (3), over-sensitivity of the patient to a well-chosen remedy and potency, one must assess the severity of the situation. What if the patient's overreaction includes pain? Constant pain quickly drains and weakens the energy of the vital force. To prevent this occurring, rapidly and calmly assess the degree to which the vital force is being depleted, so that appropriate adjunctive support may be given. Examine the patient and determine the pain tolerance level. Obtain all the information you can about the pain symptoms, all the individualizing, modifying, identifying, and characterizing features. How much is the pain troubling her? If it isn't troubling her much, let it alone to subside in its own time. If the pain is determined to be intolerable, weakening the vital force, restudy and rework the case analysis. The pain is now the most valuable symptom and is therefore used higher up in the symptom evaluation hierarchy.

In the anxiety of the moment, be very careful not to prescribe symptomatically and inadvertently induce a suppressed state on top of everything else. Restudy the case on the basis of the mental, physical, and emotional symptom *totality*, with the pain related symptoms high in the symptom hierarchy. Viewing the case in this way reduces the risk of suppression because the analysis is not based on the single, uppermost "pain" symptom in isolation from the whole person. After scientific repertory analysis and materia medica review, give the indicated remedy. Ideally, if your workings are correct, the indicated remedy should in some way relate to the previously acting remedy, decreasing the risk of suppressive homoeopathic treatment. It may be a related remedy such as an acute remedy of the constitutional (chronic) medicine, or a complementary remedy (one that completes the work of the preceding one).

This type of situation requires depth of materia medica knowledge and thorough understanding of the relationship of remedies. Many cases require a succession of remedies, administered at the appropriate intervals as indicated, each capable of taking the patient a little further along the road to cure. In order to counter

remedy overreactions, it is extremely useful to understand the sphere of operation and range of medicinal
action as well as to know how remedies are related
through their family, origin, affinities (primary sites of
action), and miasms. For instance, in an excessive, violent exacerbation of oozing, painful skin symptoms
where Sulphur has been the appropriate medicine, Hahnemann recommends Hepar Sulphuricum, which can
take the edge off the exacerbation without interfering
with the original prescription. Bearing in mind the
golden rule *never prescribe homoeopathic medicines
routinely without careful forethought,* when indicated,
Nux vomica, Phosphorus, Pulsatilla, Coffea, Chamo-
milla, and Camphora are useful remedies to consider in
cases of excessive exacerbation. Used appropriately,
they can be very effective in managing the overreaction
response. Interestingly, administration of such a related,
complementary remedy may even sometimes cure the
constitutional case altogether!

If you heed Kent's earlier comment and don't feel
confident prescribing a remedy for an overreaction
where pain is the main symptom, a mild, undynamized
analgesic may be offered. For example, in certain circumstances, aspirin could be used. This advice may
seem too radical for some purists, but pain draining the
vital force is much more detrimental to the patient than
a single dose of aspirin. Because it hasn't been dynamized or attenuated, it cannot operate on the dynamic
plane of the individual's vital force and is unlikely to
interfere with remedy action. In addition, the adjunctive
treatment gives the patient temporary relief from an
otherwise intolerable situation, and buys the practitio-

ner a little time to restudy the case. Furthermore, alleviating the pain helps the vital force to rally and get back to the job of cure.

ACTION—In evaluation (4), see scenarios 2 and 3, also treatment of oversensitive patients in Chapter 5.

9. Appearance of New Symptoms

The patient returns for follow-up and reports: "I've got new symptoms."

EVALUATION—There are several possibilities:

The patient may be experiencing symptoms of the medicine, i.e., proving the correctly chosen remedy; the patient is in a new state; or the patient is experiencing long-forgotten symptoms which have resurfaced as part of the curative process (return of old symptoms). The appearance of these old symptoms is a sign that the medicine is acting deeply in the essence of the disease. Another possibility is that the prescription was a partial one.

ACTION—Don't panic and hold on to your hat.

First of all, and this may sound silly, confirm that the patient actually took the remedy. Sometimes for a variety of reasons patients don't take the medicines suggested. If they took the medicine, check in the materia medica to see if the "new" symptoms correspond to those of the proving. If so, the prescription is a good one because the "new" symptoms are those of the medicine and in time without repetition of the dose, they will disappear of their own accord. The appearance of these

new symptoms indicates the dose has induced a proving
because the patient is hypersensitive in some degree and
therefore susceptible to overreacting to the medicine.
Hahnemann tells us in *Chronic Diseases:*

> But if the symptoms are different and had never
> before occurred, or never in this way, and,
> therefore, are peculiar to this medicine and not
> to be expected in the process of the disease, but
> trifling, the action of the medicine ought not
> for the present be interrupted. Such symptoms
> frequently pass off without interrupting the
> helpful activity of the remedy.[50]

In this case of a proving, WAIT for the symptoms to
subside before making another prescription. Also, if
you don't find the new symptoms in the proving data,
both Hahnemann and Kent say WAITING clarifies the
situation.

If the new symptoms persist:

> . . . and are of a burdensome intensity, they are
> not to be endured; in such a case they are a sign
> that the antipsoric medicine was not selected in
> the correct homoeopathic manner. Its action
> must be checked by an antidote, or when no
> antidote to it is known, another antipsoric
> medicine more accurately answering its symp-
> toms must be given in its place; in this case
> these false [new] symptoms may continue for a
> few more days, or they may return, but they
> will soon come to a final end . . .[51]

Kent explains:

> If the new symptoms decrease and the patient
> goes on to quick recovery, the new symptoms
> may in fact belong to the remedy originally pre-
> scribed, and some day be included in the prov-
> ing data of the materia medica because they are
> pathogenic symptoms. It is likely the new
> symptoms belong to that remedy but as yet
> haven't been documented in the materia med-
> ica. Some day they will fall into line as good
> symptoms to know. Keep a careful note of such
> symptoms because such watchfulness leads to
> great accuracy in prescribing as well as expan-
> sion of materia medica study.[52]

If your investigations show that the "new" symptoms are in fact long forgotten ones resurfacing, they
are a return of old symptoms, indicating the remedy is
still acting curatively. In this circumstance we must do
nothing but WAIT for the remedy to exhaust itself before giving another dose.

> If the patient has improved in regard to the
> original symptoms, and in accordance with the
> direction of cure, but now has new symptoms
> added to the remaining original ones, there has
> been a "partial" prescription.

> In this case, the remedy was selected as well as
> the symptoms of the case would allow but
> based on an indistinct symptom-picture. It has
> excited accessory symptoms and mixed some of

its own peculiar symptoms with the feelings of the patient. These accessory/new symptoms occur because they are those which the medicine is capable of producing in a particular constitution. They are only brought to light by the medicine because of its power to cause similar symptoms.[53]

Though the first remedy was inaccurately selected based on an incomplete picture, its accessory symptom inducing action serves to complete the display of the symptoms of the disease and in this way facilitates the discovery of a second, more accurate and more suitable homoeopathic medicine.[54]

In this case, Hahnemann tells us to reexamine the patient and regard the whole collection of perceptible symptoms as belonging to the disease itself, to regard the perceptible symptoms as the actual existing condition and accordingly direct treatment towards this current larger and more complete symptom group. [See *Organon,* Paragraphs 175–184 for discussion of partials in one-sided cases.][55]

If, however, after examining the patient we determine he really is experiencing *new* symptoms never ever experienced before, which do not subside, and there is no amelioration in the patient's well-being, the remedy has not acted properly and a potentially difficult situation has arisen.

Kent tells us in his tenth observation regarding new symptoms: if a great number of new symptoms appear after the administration of a remedy, the prescription will generally prove an unfavorable one. The greater the array of new symptoms coming out after the administration of a remedy, the more doubt there is thrown upon the prescription. The probability is that after these new symptoms have passed away, the patient will settle down to the original state and no improvement take place. The prescription was not homoeopathically related to the case.

According to Close, this situation indicates the first medicine was improperly selected, changing the condition of an oversensitive patient by producing new symptoms not related to the original disease and detrimental to his welfare. Discontinue the remedy and antidote with a different, better-selected one.[56]

To avoid further complications, give the patient a complete rest from medication and the symptoms should gradually subside. While waiting for things to settle down, restudy the case from the beginning, symptom by symptom. To find the right remedy and find out where you went wrong, question the patient very carefully, rework the case, and administer a better-selected remedy based on the totality of the symptom image, combining the striking new symptoms with the old ones. Put the *new* symptoms higher up in your case analysis hierarchy of characteristic symptoms, and combine the totality of the original, characteristic symptoms and the new symptoms, with more emphasis on the new symptoms.[57]

The better-selected remedy should eliminate the new symptoms and possibly modify the original symptoms. Such situations can be very difficult to manage and redirect towards cure. Unfortunately, since the first prescription was inaccurate, all subsequent prescriptions are very difficult and accompanied by great anxiety as we endeavor to unravel the muddle we have made. In this circumstance the third, fourth, fifth, and sixth prescriptions may have the same difficulties to surmount as just described. It's in dire straits like this that depth of understanding and strict adherence to Hahnemann's principles become the patient and practitioner's lifesaver. Inevitably during this time we will be testing the patient's patience!

But look on the bright side of things; it's successful management of just these very complex situations that challenges the true skill and artistry of the homoeopathic practitioner. Unraveling these muddles should encourage and inspire all of us to always give each and every case nothing less than our best shot from the start. To avert unnecessary patient suffering and practitioner confusion, we do well to heed the axiom "More Haste, Less Speed." Through consistent, meticulous case taking, accurate symptom evaluation, methodical case analysis, repertory and materia medica study, we should always aim to get the *first* prescription right.

As you proceed to right the wrong, take the pressure off yourself and discuss the situation honestly and openly with the patient, telling her why it happened and asking for her cooperation. Put yourself in your patient's shoes—wouldn't you want to know what was happening and why? When I've made mistakes, being

reminded of what Kent tells us has helped me to carry
on more effectively because it assuaged the stress.

> The patient will wait better if the doctor con-
> fesses on the spot that the selection was not
> what it ought to be, and he hopes to do better
> next time. It is a strange thing how patients will
> have an increase of confidence if the doctor will
> tell the truth. The acknowledgment of one's
> own ignorance begets confidence in an intelli-
> gent patient.[58]

Honesty between practitioner and patient enhances
integrity.

> The confidence of the patient helps the physi-
> cian to find the right remedy. His mind works
> much better when he feels he is trusted; the
> confidence of the patient sharpens his intelli-
> gence.[59]

In this stage of patient evaluation and treatment,
the Law of Similars is at work once again, in that the
dynamic action of homoeopathic medicine demands a
dynamic, crystal clear thought process from the practitioner. Hopefully, careful study of these signpost scenarios will cut through some of the most common confusing situations and clarify the various possible courses
of action to take.

In the next chapter we consider remedy responses
and case management actions for patients taking remedies in LM doses.

CHAPTER 4

1. Kent, *Minor Writings,* pg. 232.
2. Boger, *Boenninghausen's Characteristics, Materia Medica, and Repertory,* Preface, pg. 10.
3. Kent, *Lectures on Homoeopathic Philosophy,* Lecture 36, pg. 238.
4. Kent, *Lectures on Homoeopathic Philosophy,* Lecture 36, pg. 237.
5. Kent, *Lectures on Homoeopathic Philosophy,* Lecture 36, pg. 238.
6. Kent, *Lectures on Homoeopathic Philosophy,* Lecture 35, pg. 230.
7. Kent, *Minor Writings,* pg. 237.
8. Roberts, *Principles and Art of Cure by Homoeopathy,* Chapter 16, Second Prescription.
9. Kent, *Minor Writings,* pg. 234.
10. Kent, *Minor Writings,* pg. 233.
11. Farrington, *Homoeopathy and Homeopathic Prescribing,* Lesson 5, pg. 23.
12. Paraphrased from Hahnemann, *Chronic Diseases,* Volume 1, pg. 123.
13. Paraphrased from Hahnemann, *Chronic Diseases,* Volume 1, pg. 118–127.
14. Paraphrased from Hahnemann, *Chronic Diseases,* Volume 1, pg. 123.
15. See footnotes, pg. 125, *Chronic Diseases,* Volume 1.
16. Paraphrased from Hahnemann, *Chronic Diseases,* Volume 1, pg. 119–127.
17. Hahnemann, *Chronic Diseases,* Volume I, pg. 119.
18. Hahnemann, *Organon,* 6th ed. (Wesselhoeft trans.), ¶158.

19. Hahnemann, *Organon,* 6th ed. (Wesselhoeft trans.), ¶159.

20. Kent, *Lectures on Homoeopathic Philosophy,* Lecture 35, pg. 228.

21. Close, *The Genius of Homoeopathy,* Chapter 13, pg. 208.

22. Kent, *Minor Writings,* pg. 234.

23. Paraphrased from Hahnemann, *Chronic Diseases,* Volume I, pg. 119.

24. Hahnemann, *Chronic Diseases,* Volume 1, pg. 119.

25. Kent, *Lesser Writings.*

26. Schmidt, *Kent's Final General Repertory of the Homoeopathic Materia Medica,* pg. 508.

27. Hahnemann, *Organon,* 6th ed. (Boericke trans.), ¶14.

28. Kent, *Minor Writings,* pg. 314.

29. Kent, *Lectures on Homoeopathic Philosophy,* Lecture 35.

30. Kent, *Lectures on Homoeopathic Philosophy,* Lecture 35, pg. 231.

31. Wright-Hubbard, *Homoeopathy as Art and Science,* pg. 317.

32. Wright-Hubbard, *Homoeopathy as Art and Science,* pg. 317.

33. Kent, *Lectures on Homoeopathic Philosophy,* Observation No. 2.

34. Kent, *Lectures on Homoeopathic Philosophy,* Lecture 35, pg. 226 and 227.

35. Wright-Hubbard, *Homoeopathy as Art and Science,* pg. 316.

36. Close, *The Genius of Homoeopathy,* Chapter 13, pg. 207.

37. Kent, *Minor Writings,* pg. 233.

38. Close, *The Genius of Homoeopathy,* Chapter 13, pg. 207.

39. Paraphrased from Close, *The Genius of Homoeopathy,* Chapter 13, pg. 206.

40. Close, *The Genius of Homoeopathy,* Chapter 13, pg. 206.

41. Close, *The Genius of Homoeopathy,* Chapter 13, pg. 206.

42. Kent, *Minor Writings,* pg. 238.

43. Kent, *Minor Writings,* pg. 238.

44. Kent, *Minor Writings,* pg. 233.

45. Paraphrased from Hahnemann, *Chronic Diseases,* Volume 1, pg. 120.

46. Kent, *Minor Writings,* pg. 238.

47. *Paraphrases,* Volume 1, pg. 120.

48. Paraphrased from Hahnemann, *Chronic Diseases,* Volume 1, pg. 120.

49. Paraphrased from Hahnemann, *Chronic Diseases,* Volume 1, pg. 121.

50. Hahnemann, *Chronic Diseases,* Volume 1, pg. 119.

51. Hahnemann, *Chronic Diseases,* Volume 1, pg. 119.

52. Kent, *Minor Writings,* pg. 258.

53. Hahnemann, *Organon,* 6th ed. (Boericke trans.), ¶180.

54. Hahnemann, *Organon,* 6th ed. (Boericke trans.), ¶182.

55. Hahnemann, *Organon,* 6th ed. (Boericke trans.), ¶182 and 183.

56. Paraphrased from Close, *The Genius of Homoeopathy,* Chapter 13, pg. 206.

57. Paraphrased from Hahnemann, *Organon*, 6th ed. (Boericke trans.), ¶167, 179–184, Kent, *Lectures on Homoeopathic Philosophy*, Lecture 35 and Wright-Hubbard, *A Brief Study Course in Homoeopathy*, pg. 60.

58. Kent, *Lectures on Homoeopathic Philosophy*, Lecture 35, pg. 230.

59. Kent, *Lectures on Homoeopathic Philosophy*, Lecture 37, pg. 242.

CHAPTER 5

A Flexible Friend

IN THE SAME WAY MODERN pharmaceutical companies strive to reduce the adverse side effects of their medicines, so Hahnemann devoted his entire life and tireless research to developing the smallest, *least* amount of medicine necessary to effect cure. Ever the perfectionist and true scientist, Hahnemann constantly experimented with remedy dosage—potency and repetition—in order to devise the optimum method of medicine administration that could reduce or regulate the homoeopathic aggravation, and at the same time achieve the ultimate goal of *gentle,* rapid, permanent cure.

In the latter part of his research Hahnemann developed the most energetic of all homoeopathic medicines. Progressing from his original use of crude dry doses, to administering remedies in liquid form,[1] to the "plussing method" of centesimal potency administration,[2] Hahnemann finally created the LM potency—an altogether different dynamization and attenuation process described in his final version of the *Organon,* Sixth Edition.

> . . . the preparations thus produced, I have found after many laborious experiments and

counter experiments, to be the most powerful
and at the same time mildest in action, i.e., as
the most perfected.[3]

And this may be very happily effected, as recent
and oft-repeated observations have taught me,
under the following conditions: firstly, if the
medicine selected with the utmost care was per-
fectly homoeopathic; secondly, if it is highly
potentized, dissolved in water, and given in a
proper small dose in definite intervals that experience has taught is the most suitable for the
quickest accomplishment of the cure but with
the precaution, *that the degree of every dose
deviate somewhat from the preceding and following* in order that the vital principle which is
to be altered to a similar medicinal disease be
not aroused to untoward reactions and revolt
as is always the case with unmodified and especially rapidly repeated doses.[4]

But during the last four or five years, however,
all these difficulties are wholly solved by my
new altered but perfected method. The same
carefully selected medicine may now be given
daily and for months, if necessary in this way,
namely, after the lower degree of potency has
been used for one or two weeks in the treatment of chronic disease, advance is made in the
same way to higher degrees, (beginning according to the new dynamization method, taught
herewith with the use of the lowest degrees).[5]

But if the succeeding dose is changed slightly every time, namely potentized somewhat higher, then the vital principle may be altered without difficulty by the same medicine (the sensation of natural disease diminishing) and thus the cure brought nearer.[6]

In taking one and the same medicine repeatedly (which is indispensable to secure the cure of a serious/chronic disease) if the dose is in every case varied and modified only a little in its degree of dynamization, then the vital force of the patient will calmly, and as it were willingly receive the same medicine even at brief intervals very many times in succession with the best results, every time increasing the well-being of the patient.[7]

Because the sixth edition of the *Organon* remained unpublished until 1921, great homoeopaths of the past such as Kent never saw it and therefore practiced their healing art without knowledge of the LM potency. Only recently have the LMs become more generally available from homoeopathic pharmacies. Most modern homoeopaths still prescribe only decimal or centesimal potencies, either because they haven't understood that certain paragraphs of the sixth edition relate in large part to LMs (¶246, 248, 252, 253, 256, 257, 273, and 277 through 283),* or because there is confusion concern-

---

* There is also a lot of inappropriate, repeated dosing of decimal and centesimal potencies due to a misunderstanding of these paragraphs that refer to LM potencies only.

ing their effective use. (Preparation, administration, and evaluation of remedy action are more involved with LM doses.)

Every educated homoeopath knows that in order to regulate and minimize any initial aggravations, the skill and art of successful homoeopathy must include not only the selection of the right remedy, but also the selection of the appropriate dosage. In addition, homoeopaths must know how frequently a dose should be administered in order to speed the patient toward restoration of balance and health. Those who use the LM potency know it is particularly effective in a wide range of complex disorders where an aggravation of any kind, no matter how slight or fleeting, must be avoided.

Some instances in which LM administration would be appropriate are as follows:

• Individuals suffering chronic, deep-seated disorders, e.g., chronic fatigue syndrome, multiple sclerosis, cancer, AIDS.

• Palliation of incurable states.

• Very low vitality or lack of reaction.

• Complex skin disorders such as eczema, psoriasis, and inveterate acne.

• Treatment of individuals concurrently taking allopathic medication as with high blood pressure or diabetes, etc.

• Management of individuals with recurrent acute exacerbation of the chronic case, i.e., asthma, epilepsy, etc.

• Alcohol or drug abuse.

• A history of symptoms suppressed by long-term, multiple, allopathic medical regimens.

• Individuals who are hypersensitive to their environments and therefore very sensitive to remedies, e.g., chemical sensitivity disorders. Or individuals needlessly rendered hypersensitive by too many and too high doses of homoeopathic medicines due to lack of understanding about utilization of potentiation scales.

• Deep mental troubles.

Individuals suffering these and many other complicated imbalances may benefit tremendously from administration of LM potencies.

Of course, over-stimulation of the vital force may be effectively reduced by using the *plussing* administration method of centesimal potencies.[8] However, the remarkable range of therapeutic action derived from the LM potency expands the *gentle,* curative potential of modern homoeopathic practice even further. Although centesimal potencies generally act more rapidly than LMs in acute illness, LMs may be used in both acute and chronic states. Their obvious flexibility and curative power means some practitioners use LMs almost exclusively.

However, it is essential to emphasize, as in all homoeopathic treatment, because its success lies in symptom image individualization, nothing should be done routinely. Authentic homoeopathy views each individual and his symptoms as a completely unique case. Neither medicine nor potency selection is based on anything less than the *individuality* and *totality* of symptom image of each case, as manifest in the perceived strange, rare, and peculiar characteristic symptoms, experienced by each individual in that particular state of distress. For example, no matter how many cases of eczema we have resolved in the past using a particular potency or remedy, to know what is the most appropriate dose, the most suitable degree of minuteness for sure and gentle remedial effect, each patient's particular state of imbalance must be viewed as a unique set of circumstances requiring an individualized treatment program. As Hahnemann teaches:

> . . . to determine for every particular medicine, what dose of it will suffice for homoeopathic therapeutic purposes and yet be so minute that the gentlest and most rapid cure may be thereby obtained [is] not the work of theoretical speculation, not by finespun reasoning, not by specious sophistry [theorizing] . . . It is just as impossible as to tabulate in advance all imaginable cases. Pure experiment, careful observation of the sensitiveness of each patient, and accurate experience can alone determine this *in each individual case.*[9]

Preparation and Administration of LM Potencies

Since LM potencies were not widely used at the time of the early great homoeopaths, their literature offers no guidance on the subject. Having researched the subject in Hahnemann's writings and information from homoeopathic pharmacists in the United Kingdom and the United States, I have come to understand the following about LM use:

The homoeopath purchases LM potentized gran-
ules from a reliable homoeopathic pharmacy, one that
prepares LMs strictly according to Hahnemann's instructions in the *Organon*. The homoeopath then
makes up the medicine stock bottle for the patient by
crushing one granule of the LM 1 (01) with a few grains
of sugar of milk (saclac) in forty, thirty, twenty, fifteen,
or eight tablespoons of water, and 2 or 3 drops of alcohol to preserve it.[10] (It is thought the variations in number of tablespoons of water relate to the length of time
the stock bottle will last.) For practical purposes, Hahnemann recommended dissolving the LM granule in 7
to 8 tablespoons of water, succussing it, then pouring
one tablespoon of this liquid into a glass containing a
further 7 to 8 tablespoons of water. To slightly increase
the degree of dynamization, this is then stirred thoroughly and a teaspoonful dose is given to the patient.
At the beginning of each day's dosing, the patient gives
the medicine stock bottle eight to twelve succussions, by
striking it against something firm yet yielding such as
the palm of one's hand or, in Hahnemann's fashion, a
"leather-bound book."

Hahnemann gives a wide range of possible dilutions. However, for ease of administration, in the
United States, the stock bottle is usually prepared in either a four- or an eight-ounce bottle and in the United
Kingdom, generally in a 110 or 160 ml. bottle.

From the stock bottle the patient then pours one
tablespoonful of the liquid into a small glass or jar containing 7 to 8 tablespoonfuls of water, and stirs or
shakes this mixture thoroughly. One teaspoonful is then
taken as the first dose.

As needed, several teaspoonful doses may be taken through the day with succussions of the jar between each dose. *A fresh solution must be prepared from the stock bottle daily.* The jar is rinsed with hot water, then cooled before preparing the new dilution as described above.

> [A] slight change in the degree of dynamization is . . . effected, if the bottle, which contains the solution of one or more pellets is merely shaken five or six times, every time before taking it . . . if the dose is in every case varied and modified only a little in its degree of dynamization, then the vital force of the patient will calmly, and as it were, willingly receive *the same* medicine even at brief intervals very many times in succession with the best results, every time increasing the well-being of the patient.[11]

In this way, each dose of the LM medicine stimulates a slight, almost imperceptible, reaction from the vital force, taking the patient gently, rung by rung up the ladder of cure toward restoration of health.

Dosing regimens vary according to the patient's state. In acute cases, doses may be repeated every two, three, four, or six hours. In very urgent cases or emergency situations, doses may be repeated every hour or more frequently. In chronic conditions, doses may be taken daily, every second day or as often as needed. If many doses are needed in one day, a new solution is prepared, as described above, when the jar is empty. In determining the dosage we must as always bear in mind Hahnemann's principle of the minimum dose, as it refers not only to potency but also to frequency. The optimum dose is the minimum dose required to effect cure.

Providing the patient improves according to the Law of Cure, without experiencing new symptoms, this dosing method may be repeated for months with ever increasing success.

As you would expect, dosage frequency or duration of administration is never prescribed routinely. Lack of reaction cases may need more stimulation while oversensitive ones require less. As treatment continues the patient may need the remedy more or less frequently. Our guide is always the state of the vital force.

By varying quantity and succussions—the size and number of spoonfuls taken and strikes given to the stock bottle—we are able to manipulate the dosage very precisely matching the unique individual character of the disturbance, in tandem with the pace of the patient's vital force, and its state of disease. It may be necessary to give more teaspoonfuls (larger doses) and/or more succussive strikes (for instance, twelve succussions of the stock bottle gives a slightly sharper daily rise in potency than eight), in order to take the patient faster up the potency scale towards cure.

It's extremely important to emphasize that frequency and quantity of dosing must always reflect the level of each individual's sensitivity and susceptibility to the medicine. There are patients who are a thousand times more sensitive than the least sensitive patients. For those in whom we see considerable sensitivity, doses should be increased far more slowly and by far smaller amounts than for patients who are less sensitive, for whom doses can be more rapidly increased.[12] If you are treating an unusually sensitive individual, a teaspoonful of diluted liquid from the dosing glass or jar may be put in a second jar of water, thoroughly stirred, and doses of a teaspoonful or more can be taken from the second glass or jar. This is commonly termed "double diluting" and is typically employed in cases where the patient experiences or is perceived to run the risk of experiencing an overreaction to the medicine, as often happens in hypersensitive individuals. To minimize aggravations, such patients may require a third or even fourth jar to be similarly prepared.[13] This double/triple/quadruple dilution decision is made on the basis of the patient's carefully monitored self-experimentation with the remedy.

If the solution is used up, and if the same medicine is still indicated, it is necessary to add to the next stock bottle solution one or (rarely) several pellets of a higher potency (the next in sequence, LM2), with which we continue so long as the patient experiences continued improvement.[14] In other words, as long as the patient improves, when the end of a stock bottle of one potency is reached, the patient moves on to the stock bottle of the next higher potency, dosing according to need in the usual manner. To avoid giving the wrong potency at the wrong time and interrupting the curative process, always begin dosing with LM 1 (01) potency and move up through the potencies in sequential order.

Interpreting the Patient's Response to the LM Potency

The patient begins taking a dose of one or several teaspoonfuls daily or every other day as appropriate. As the LMs have a different pattern of patient response from centesimals, it is advisable in the beginning to monitor patient progress very carefully. Patients should initially check in with the practitioner every five days.

1. Amelioration Without Aggravation

At check-in, the patient reports improvement with no aggravation. There are no troublesome complaints or new symptoms.

EVALUATION—The remedy is acting.

ACTION—Dosing continues up through the scale so long as the patient improves steadily.[15] Check in with the patient may be extended to 10 or 14 days.

2. Continued Amelioration with Eventual Return of Presenting Symptoms

All goes well. The patient modifies the dose each time by succussion. The patient continues dosing until, while feeling generally better, she begins once again to experience one or more of the original, presenting symptoms in a mild to moderate degree.[16]

EVALUATION—The artificial disease (the remedy), so similar to the natural disease (presenting symptoms), is now almost the only one acting.[17] This return of presenting symptoms indicates that cure is imminent, and that in order to stop experiencing the natural disease, the vital principle has almost no more need to be affected by the similar, medicinal disease.[18] This indicates that the life principle, now free of the natural disease, is beginning to suffer somewhat from an excess of homoeopathic medicine.[19] In other words the patient is now experiencing the homoeopathic aggravation, as it were, at the end of treatment.[20]

Note carefully: under the influence of LM potencies, the timing of the appearance of the homoeopathic
aggravation is different from that of centesimals. (The
centesimal homoeopathic excitation, if it occurs, is expected to appear at the *beginning* of treatment.)

ACTION—To be convinced of the fact that cure is imminent, the patient should discontinue dosing for a week
or two. If the symptoms experienced are those of the
homoeopathic medicinal disease, (if they are due to excess remedy, the symptoms of the remedy mimicking the
natural disease), they will disappear within a few hours
or days during this interval off the medicine, leaving un-
clouded health in their wake.[21] Provided the patient
continues the recommended lifestyle changes, no more
symptoms will manifest and in all probability the patient will be cured.[22]

3. Remnants of the Disease Persist after Treatment

What happens if on the other hand, at the end of
this period without medicine, remnants of the previously observed disease (presenting symptoms) are still
manifesting?[23]

EVALUATION—This indicates that the original disease
has not yet been completely extinguished. Traces of the
original complaint remain.[24]

ACTION—To advance the patient toward cure, treatment with higher potencies must be renewed.[25] In other
words, dosing should be continued from where it was
left off.

4. No Amelioration Occurs

After a few days on the LM 1 (01), there is no improvement in the patient at all.

EVALUATION—There are three possible reasons for this situation:

(1) The remedy is incorrectly selected.

(2) There is a block in the action of the remedy due to some environmental or maintaining cause that is preventing curative progress.[26]

(3) There is lack of reaction in the vital force.

ACTION (3)—Try igniting a spark of activity by increasing the frequency of doses. If the remedy still fails to act, discontinue dosing, and carefully restudy the case for errors. If an error in analysis is found, rework the case and administer the better-selected remedy. If, after progressively increasing the dose, a different set of symptoms is experienced, this is an unfavorable response and another, more appropriate remedy must be found.

ACTION (2)—You determine the first remedy to be the correct one, and the remedy has not acted due to a maintaining cause. Remember, to bring about permanent cure, maintaining causes must first of all be removed. Before considering any further remedy administration, discuss the situation with the patient and develop appropriate strategies for removing the maintaining cause. At the appropriate time, administer the indicated remedy. If, after restudying the case, the same remedy is indicated and the maintaining cause is removed, the remedy should now act and the patient will begin to improve. If this does not occur, either there is an error in your understanding of the case and remedy choice, or the case may be incurable. If the maintaining cause cannot be removed for some reason, it becomes an obstacle to cure. Treatment proceeds but full recovery is obviously hampered.

ACTION (1)—In this circumstance, search for a better indicated remedy.[27]

5. Intensification of Symptoms at Beginning of Treatment

At *commencement of treatment,* after only a few days on the remedy, the originally observed symptoms are intensified and the patient feels worse in any respect.[28]

EVALUATION—A homoeopathic aggravation has occurred at the beginning of treatment. Either the dose is too large and the patient's vital force is overstimulated, or the medicine was inaccurately selected. Such an intensification of the original symptoms of chronic disease should appear only at the end of treatment when cure is almost or completely finished.[29]

ACTION—The dose must be reduced.[30] Stop the remedy to see if the symptoms subside of their own accord and do not recur. If this happens, it means the patient needs no further medicine. If after a day or two off the remedy the original symptoms continue at the intensified level, the patient may alleviate the aggravation by adopting the LM administration method for sensitive patients, as described previously and in the footnote to the *Organon*, Paragraph 248.[31]

If the aggravated symptoms persist after trying multiple dilutions, then the remedy must be incorrect. Dosing is discontinued while a more appropriate remedy is selected after restudying the case.[32]

Alternatively, dosing can be reduced by extending the intervals between each dose or by preparing the daily dose with half a tablespoonful instead of a full tablespoonful from the stock bottle. Since homoeopathy is about treating the individual nature of each patient, it is appropriate that in the LM administration method, alleviating the homoeopathic aggravation is now directly under the control of the patient who is invited to experiment with manipulating the dose to find the frequency and size of dose most suitable to effect cure without causing discomfort.

6. *New Symptoms Appear*

The patient commences dosing and continues as long as there is steady improvement and no appearance of any significant new symptoms, never experienced before. Then one day the patient reports one or another complaint he never had before.

EVALUATION—The disease image has changed. It is now manifesting in a group of altered, new symptoms. A medicine which, in the course of its action, produces new and troublesome symptoms not pertaining to the disease to be cured is not capable of effecting real improvement and cannot be considered homoeopathically selected.[33] When there is not even a slight improvement or an aggravation it is incorrect and likely harmful to repeat or increase the dose in the mistaken belief that it is too small to act effectively.[34] In cases where there has been no significant change in the patient's lifestyle, nor any event affecting the emotions, yet new symptoms appear during treatment, the remedy is invariably incorrect. It never indicates the dose has been too small.

ACTION—Whether the new symptoms are violent or not, order must be reestablished as quickly as possible. The medicine must be replaced with another, more homoeopathic one that accurately reflects the new state of the disease.[35] Administer the new remedy in the same, repeated doses, mindful before each dose to gradually modify and increase its potency with thorough, vigorous succussions.[36]

Like many others, I was originally shy of using LM potencies because of the apparent difficulty in their case management. Now, since restudying Hahnemann and others on the subject, I am enthusiastic about administering them in the appropriate circumstances. Their proper use opens a door to wonderful results in otherwise very difficult cases.

The real beauty and curative potential of LM potencies is their infinite flexibility. The dose can be precisely manipulated by patients themselves to meet their particular and individual needs. With patients in control of their own curative process, what better way could there be to tap into the body's self-healing mechanism and restore health rapidly, gently, and (where possible) permanently?

CHAPTER 5

1. Hahnemann, *Organon,* 5th and 6th ed. (Dudgeon trans.), ¶286.

2. Hahnemann, *Chronic Diseases,* Volume 1, pg. 156.

3. Hahnemann, *Organon,* 6th ed. (Boericke trans.), footnote 156 to ¶270.

4. Hahnemann, *Organon,* 6th ed. (Boericke trans.), ¶246.

5. Hahnemann, *Organon,* 6th ed. (Boericke trans.), footnote 132 to ¶246.

6. Hahnemann, *Organon,* 6th ed. (Boericke trans.), ¶247.

7. Hahnemann, *Chronic Diseases,* Volume 1, pg. 156.

8. Hahnemann, *Chronic Diseases,* Volume 1, pg. 156.

9. Hahnemann, *Organon,* 6th ed. (Boericke trans.), ¶278.

10. Hahnemann, *Organon,* 6th ed. (Boericke trans.), ¶248 and footnote.

11. Hahnemann, *Chronic Diseases,* Volume 1, pg. 156.

12. Hahnemann, *Organon,* 6th ed. (Boericke trans.), ¶281.

13. Hahnemann, *Organon,* 6th ed. (Boericke trans.), footnote to ¶248.

14. Hahnemann, *Organon,* 6th ed. (Boericke trans.), ¶248.

15. Hahnemann, *Organon,* 6th ed. (Boericke trans.), ¶280.

16. Hahnemann, *Organon,* 6th ed. (Boericke trans.), ¶280.

17. Hahnemann, *Organon,* 6th ed. (Boericke trans.), ¶248.

18. Hahnemann, *Organon,* 6th ed. (Boericke trans.), ¶148.

19. Hahnemann, *Organon,* 6th ed. (Boericke trans.), ¶248, 280.

20. Hahnemann, *Organon,* 6th ed. (Boericke trans.), ¶161, 280.

21. Hahnemann, *Organon,* 6th ed. (Boericke trans.), ¶248, 281.

22. Hahnemann, *Organon,* 6th ed. (Boericke trans.), ¶281.

23. Hahnemann, *Organon,* 6th ed. (Boericke trans.), ¶281.

24. Hahnemann, *Organon,* 6th ed. (Boericke trans.), ¶281.

25. Hahnemann, *Organon,* 6th ed. (Boericke trans.), ¶281.

26. Hahnemann, *Organon,* 6th ed. (Boericke trans.), ¶252.

27. Hahnemann, *Organon,* 6th ed. (Boericke trans.), ¶248, 256.

28. Hahnemann, *Organon,* 6th ed. (Boericke trans.), ¶282.

29. Hahnemann, *Organon,* 6th ed. (Boericke trans.), ¶161.

30. Hahnemann, *Organon,* 6th ed. (Boericke trans.), ¶282.

31. Hahnemann, *Organon,* 6th ed. (Boericke trans.), ¶248.

32. Hahnemann, *Organon,* 6th ed. (Boericke trans.), ¶283.

33. Hahnemann, *Organon,* 6th ed. (Boericke trans.), ¶249.

34. Hahnemann, *Organon,* 6th ed. (Boericke trans.), footnote to ¶249.

35. Hahnemann, *Organon,* 6th ed. (Boericke trans.), ¶167.

36. Hahnemann, *Organon,* 6th ed. (Boericke trans.), ¶248–250.

CHAPTER 6

When To Change the Remedy

Now for the biggest bugaboo in homoeopathic practice: Is it time to try another remedy?

Generally, the chief obstacles to making a successful second prescription are the desire for a rapid cure and ignorance about when to change the remedy. It is after the first prescription that we are at greatest risk of making the *three worst mistakes* defined by Hahnemann as follows:

> The first is to consider the dose too small to act. The second, the chief error in the cure of chronic diseases, is to make the wrong choice of remedy through inexactness, lack of earnestness, and love of ease. The third leading mistake, which we cannot too carefully, steadfastly avoid, is in hastily, thoughtlessly, giving some other medicine in the mistaken supposition that so small a dose couldn't possibly operate for more than eight or ten days.[1]

In essence, the second prescription is all about *timing*. In tackling the thorny issue of changing the remedy, Kent offers some clear guidelines:

> To change to the next remedy becomes a ponderous problem, and what shall it be? *The last*

appearing symptom shall be the guide to the next remedy. This is so whenever the image has been permitted to settle by watching and waiting for the shaping of the returning symptom picture. Long have I waited after exhausting the power of the remedy, while observing a few of the old [presenting] symptoms returning; finally a new symptom appears. This latest symptom will appear in the anamnesis* as best related to some medicine having it as a characteristic, which most likely has all the rest of the symptoms. It is not supposed that this later appearing symptom is an old symptom on its way to final departure, for so long as old symptoms reappear and disappear it is granted that no medicine is to be thought of[2] . . . it is an error to think of a medicine when a symptom–image is changing. The physician must wait for permanency or firmness in the relations of the image before making a prescription.[3]

Before changing remedies, Kent cautions us to wait for a clear image to emerge. If the symptom picture represents a return of old symptoms, the same remedy and slightly modified potency is all that is required. The time to think of changing the remedy is when truly new symptoms appear and settle firmly and permanently, indicating a new symptom picture has come in view. Then we find:

---

* Anamnesis: a recalling to mind; recollection.

A second prescription is sometimes necessary
to complement the former and this is always a
change of remedy.[4]

Kent gives the example of complementary remedies
with a patient relieved by Belladonna to some degree,
but then needing the constitutional remedy, Calcarea,
which is the chronic remedy of Belladonna. He also discusses the usefulness of related remedies called for in a
series.

A medicine always leads to one of its cognates
and we find that the cognates are closely related to each other . . .[5]

The new symptom image will call for a related remedy. In his *Lectures*, Kent advises us to change the remedy when the treatment plan changes. For example,
your opening plan of treatment assumes the case is
psoric in nature because all the symptoms in the case
and case history indicate the psoric miasm. You have
given antipsoric medicines, the patient did very well,
and the psoric symptoms have disappeared. Then the
patient presents with an ulcerated sore throat and a severe headache; an old syphilitic condition has come up.
You adjust your treatment to this new state of affairs.
When one miasm is uppermost, the other is quiet. You
change your treatment plan according to the state of the
patient.[6]

This advice is particularly relevant in managing
patients experiencing *alternating states,* which ideally
would indicate a remedy that covers the alternation, or
might require a succession of related remedies. The na-

ture of alternating states makes them complicated to manage successfully. They require a deep understanding of homoeopathic philosophy.

Too large a topic to tackle here, suffice to say alternating states occur for a variety of reasons. Primarily they arise due to a complexity and alternation of prevailing miasms; the alternating action of some medicines, e.g., Ignatia; the nature of the progression of disease and the subsequent reaction of the vital force. Interactions between these three forces result in alternating states. Interested readers will find the bulk of Hahnemann's instructions on the management of alternating states in the *Organon* and Volume 1 of *Chronic Diseases.*

Although as stated, we adapt our treatment plan to the state of the patient, Kent advises *against changing the remedy when the symptoms change only slightly.*

> While watching the prescriptions of beginners, I have observed very often the proper results of the first prescription. The patient has improved for a time, then ceased to respond to any remedy. Close investigation generally reveals that this patient improved after the first dose of medicine, that the symptoms changed slightly without new symptoms, and the new "photo" seemed to call for some other remedy, the remedy was changed and trouble began. Constant changing of remedies followed until all the antipsorics in *Chronic Diseases* had been given on flitting symptom-images, and the patient is yet sick. This is the common experience of

young Hahnemannians trying to find the right way.[7]

The golden rule is never, ever change a remedy without a very good reason.

So when exactly do we change the remedy?

Apart from when we observe *no change* in the presenting symptom-image after administering a remedy, it is time for a new remedy when striking new symptoms appear and there is a clear change in the symptom picture upon which you based your first prescription. For instance, perhaps the headache that has lasted a long time disappears, or the patient's depression has gone and in exchange a new group of symptoms appears somewhere in the body, such as the patient never had before. At this time, a new remedy must be considered because there is a change of state in the disturbance and a new symptom image has emerged. Under such circumstances the case calls for a change of remedy. Only change the remedy if the symptoms have changed, perhaps revealing a different miasmatic state. But while the patient is improving even though they may still experience some remaining (original) symptoms, don't touch it. Leave the remedy alone to complete its curative action.

> So long as curative action can be obtained, and even though the symptoms have changed, provided the patient is improving, hands off. Whenever in doubt, wait. It is a rule, after you have gone through a series of potencies, never to leave that remedy until one or more doses of

a higher potency have been given and tested. But when this dose of a higher potency has been given and tested without effect . . . a change is necessary.[8]

Never, ever change the remedy if the patient has improved. Before deserting a well-indicated, well-selected remedy and switching to another, try a higher potency. If you have exhausted the ascending scale try starting again at the potency you originally gave the patient before giving up on a well-indicated remedy. As stated before, patients respond differently to the same potency, because the vital force is in a different state of health the second time around.

Situations Calling for a New Remedy

Suggested approaches to treatment of different kinds of clinical situations where a new remedy is called for are discussed below.

1. Curative Action Followed by Change in Picture

After the first prescription there has been an amelioration of symptoms and continued improvement for two or three ascending potencies. The next dose is given, after which there is no reaction to the medicine, no improvement, and no change in the symptoms, except for the appearance of a symptom not previously mentioned by the patient.

EVALUATION—Up until the last dose the remedy has acted and has now stopped acting. The appearance of a "new" symptom at this stage is often an indication that perhaps at the time of the original case working this particular information was not available and consequently the first case analysis did not cover the complete totality of the individual's suffering. In other words the first medicine matched only part of the disorder picture and not the whole. Since the selected medicine was not similar enough to cover the whole totality, it was unable to hold the case through a series of potencies and bring about complete cure. To complete cure, patients often require a series of carefully selected remedies, administered as indicated, one remedy at a time over a period of time

ACTION—Retake the case and look for a new remedy that more accurately resembles the new symptom image. Be careful to ensure that the new symptom declared is not, in fact, a return of an old symptom. Examine the patient closely. You may discover she has suffered this symptom in the past but forgotten to mention it. On the other hand, if examination reveals new information, it's necessary to restudy the case and seek another remedy that better reflects the current changed symptom image totality.

> After administration of the new, well-chosen medicine, the patient will say, "This new remedy acted like the first one did in the beginning." Patients feel the medicine when it is acting, working properly.[9]

2. Symptoms Worsen

At the follow-up the patient says, "I'm much worse in every respect." You go through the case in detail with him to ascertain if this is true on the mental, emotional, and physical levels.

EVALUATION—On the face of it, it looks like a bad sign. There has been no amelioration. There is a steady worsening of all symptoms, and the disease is progressing inwards, in the wrong Direction of Cure. Be careful.

This bad response may be due to one of several possibilities: (1) the wrong remedy; (2) the correct remedy, but wrong potency, chosen because of incorrect perception of the state of the patient's vital force, susceptibility, and miasms; (3) the right remedy, whose curative effect is blocked by a miasmatic barrier; or (4) the true picture of the inner disturbance was masked by the effects of allopathic drugs and you were unable, at the outset, to accurately perceive the symptom image totality. If in the latter case, the patient under homoeopathic treatment (and monitored by his allopathic physician), has safely and gradually withdrawn from the allopathic drugs, then the vital force, like an escaped prisoner, will respond to release from suppressive treatment by enthusiastically exercising its newfound freedom. In true curative fashion, it vigorously exteriorizes the previously suppressed disturbance, providing a different symptom picture representing the patient's state as it was *before* suppressive treatment.

ACTION—If the patient's symptoms are severe, they demand rapid action without delay. Restudy the case according to the new symptom image and find the correct potency and remedy. If your new case analysis brings you to the same remedy, before prescribing, examine your workings carefully for concrete, supportive evidence. Consult the materia medica for confirmatory symptoms and if you are confident in the accuracy of your analysis, give the medicine and potency indicated. This is a typical situation in which the LM potency might be most helpful. (See Chapter 5.)

If the aggravation is less severe, WAIT. Attentively monitor the patient's progress regularly and at short intervals. Wait for the true disease image to emerge clearly, then retake the case, and give the better-indicated remedy or potency.

ACTION FOR POSSIBILITY (1)—If you conclude the wrong remedy was administered, examine the patient carefully, restudy the case for errors, rectify them, and select a better-indicated medicine.

ACTION FOR POSSIBILITY (2)—If you gave the wrong potency, restudy the case to determine the state of the patient's vital force and susceptibility, the degree of predominant miasmatic activity, and administer a more appropriate potency.

ACTION FOR POSSIBILITY (3)—If you determine that there is a miasmatic barrier in the case, retake the case and analyze it according to the persisting symptoms. Select a more miasmatically appropriate remedy, which by its nature goes deeper into the case, or if indicated (if the patient's symptom picture corresponds to the provings), to break through the miasmatic barrier, give a nosode that reflects the uppermost miasm(s).

3. *Aggravation with Brief Interval of Amelioration*

The patient says: "I've been worse, except for 4 or 5 days of feeling better, then I got worse again."

EVALUATION—This is a prolonged aggravation, better briefly, then worse again. There was a quick, short amelioration of 4 or 5 days followed by a relapse to the original or a worse condition. This relapsing state may indicate a partial remedy or possibly a nearly incurable case with severe pathology and a poor prognosis.

> This may be because the remedy was only partly similar, or insufficient as to dosage; but where this occurrence is observed several times in succession and lasting improvement does not follow carefully selected remedies, it means that the case is incurable. There is not vitality enough to sustain a curative reaction, and dissolution is imminent.[10]

ACTION—The seriousness of the situation dictates that treatment proceed with utmost caution. Calmly and methodically apply logical case analysis. Search for the new remedy, reflecting the symptom image totality of the relapsing state. If you perceive the same symptom image totality, the vital force is calling for the same remedy. Repeat the remedy at a higher potency or give the LM potency, which is more appropriate for relapsing cases with serious pathology.

Challenging situations like this demand considerable time and attention and frequent patient reports. If the remedy image is unclear, and the patient can tolerate her condition, suspend medication. Watch and wait actively for a clearer symptom picture to emerge, indicating a different remedy.

I have always found the decision of when to change the remedy a very difficult one. My inhibited, psoric heart is always in my mouth! Only after administering the new remedy and seeing the patient continue along the curative path, do I ever completely relax in the logic of this wonderful healing system.

A quick review of this chapter reveals frequent repetition of the precaution WAIT. Chapter 8 discusses the whys and wherefores of the art of waiting. Waiting may often be the most difficult thing for both patient and practitioner to do, but it reaps unparalleled rewards.

CHAPTER 6

1. Paraphrased from Hahnemann *Chronic Diseases,* Volume I, pg. 120–122.
2. Kent, *Lesser Writings,* pg. 419.
3. Kent, *Minor Writings,* pg. 234.
4. Kent, *Lectures on Homoeopathic Philosophy,* Lecture 36, pg. 240.
5. Kent, *Lectures on Homoeopathic Philosophy,* Lecture 36, pg. 240.
6. Kent, *Lectures on Homoeopathic Philosophy,* Lecture 36, pg. 241.
7. Kent, *Minor Writings,* pg. 236.
8. Kent, *Lectures on Homoeopathic Philosophy,* Lecture 36, pg. 240.
9. Kent, *Lesser Writings,* pg. 208.
10. Close, *The Genius of Homoeopathy,* Chapter 13, pg. 208.

CHAPTER 7

Golden Rules

This chapter provides essential rules of the road to rapid recovery gleaned from my research. In resolving difficult situations, they have proved to be extremely effective guidelines for successful case management.

• Always avoid haste.

• No prescription can be made for any patient, except after careful and prolonged study of the case, to know what it promises in the symptoms, and everything that has existed previously.[1]

You may be caught unaware by an unanticipated explosion of an unexpected miasm and not know what is happening, or what to do to salvage the situation, therefore:

• Do not administer a medicine without knowing the constitution of the patient, because it is a hazardous and dangerous thing to do.[2]

• Unless the LM is administered, always prescribe a single dose and wait for the response of the vital force before prescribing again.

• For clearest instructions on the correct action/direction to take, observe and be guided by the state of the vital force as expressed in the appearance, disappearance, and reappearance of symptoms.

- Before prescribing again, wait long enough for original (presenting) symptoms to return. Wait for the same image to return, which is the vital force calling for the same remedy.

- When the presenting symptoms return unchanged or diminished in frequency, duration, and intensity, the remedy selection is correct.

- Watch and wait. The reflex action of all prescribers should be to wait.

- Never prescribe for a moving target. Wait until the symptom image has settled and is clear.

- Waiting must be governed by knowledge. To know waiting is right is quite different from waiting without a fixed purpose.[3]

- There is no fixed time for waiting. Depending on the state of the individual's vital force and the nature of the disturbance experienced, it may be years, months, weeks, days, or minutes.

- The length of time is not so important as being on the safe side, and waiting is the only safe thing to do.[4]

- Never desert a remedy that has acted curatively until, after proceeding through ascending potencies, you are certain the remedy has exhausted its curative action and a truly new symptom image has appeared.

- When the picture comes back unaltered, except by the absence of one or more presenting symptoms, the remedy should never be changed.

- Go to the next highest potency when the previous one is exhausted.

- *If in doubt, wait.* Reexamine the case to assure yourself of the accuracy of your previous prescription.

- Avoid premature prescriptions and interference with the curative action of the vital force.

- Never prescribe more than one remedy at once. You won't know which one has acted or why, or how to follow the preceding prescription.

- Honesty is the best policy. If you make a mistake, declare it to yourself and your patient.

- Refuse to act impulsively, routinely, or in a panic. In the second prescription, you'll always do good work if you go on the premise that the vital force will tell us, through the symptoms, what it needs

- Observe before you decide, think before you act.

I conclude this chapter with statements from Kent and Hahnemann that encapsulate much of what is needed to make the second prescription, quoting first from Dr. Pierre Schmidt's biography of Kent in *Kent's Final General Repertory.*

> Kent used to give his students two bits of advice among others, which I would like to recall here, for they were transmitted to me by his most intimate disciples, Dr. Austin and Dr. Gladwin: "When you have prescribed one, two, three remedies, especially in acute cases, but of course also in chronic cases, without results, I beg you stop, do not continue. This is the moment to give *Placebo,* which you should have done at the beginning, to good effect. Applying this rule is much more difficult than just

'doing something' by giving a badly chosen remedy of which you're not sure, and which does not correspond to the essential symptoms of the case, either because you do not know the remedy, or because you do not know the patient's essential symptoms.

Don't give any remedy before reconsidering your case; patiently await the development of symptoms, like a hunter stalking his prey and waiting until it is properly visible to fire the shot which will kill it. Learn how to wait and observe, and don't lose your head."[5]

Quoting from the same source, this is Kent's second piece of advice:

"Every time you study a case to find the constitutional remedy, don't simply limit yourself to finding the *simillimum* (the remedy with the most qualitative and quantitative similarity), but like William Tell, who was commanded to shoot an arrow into an apple resting on his son's head, and selected two arrows instead of one (the second for the man who had given him the order, if he missed the mark and hit his son), always have a second remedy up your sleeve, a remedy as much as possible similar to the first; in this way you will not be at a loss for your second prescription."[6]

Next, we turn to Dr. Hahnemann for further words of wisdom: while improvement still perceptibly progresses it is a fundamental rule in treatment of chronic diseases to let the action of the remedy come to an undisturbed conclusion so long as it visibly advances the cure. This method forbids any new prescription, any interruption by another medicine, and forbids as well the immediate repetition of the same remedy.[7]

In other words, never repeat a medicine while improvement continues and the remedy is still acting. Continuing with Hahnemann's advice:

> Homoeopaths should not allow a new dose of a medicine to be taken or given without convincing ourselves in every case beforehand as to its usefulness. The only allowable exception to the rule is when the dose of a well-selected, beneficial remedy has made some beginning toward improvement, but its action ceases too quickly, its power is too soon exhausted, and the cure does not proceed any further.[8]

CHAPTER 7

1. Kent, *Lectures on Homoeopathic Philosophy,* Lecture 36, pg. 241.
2. Kent, *Lectures on Homoeopathic Philosophy,* Lecture 36, pg. 241.
3. Kent, *Minor Writings, The Second Prescription—* Paraphrased.
4. Kent, *Minor Writings, The Second Prescription—* Paraphrased.
5. Schmidt, *Kent's Final General Repertory,* P. Schmidt, ed., pg. 7.

6. Schmidt, *Kent's Final General Repertory,* P. Schmidt, ed., pg. 7.

7. Paraphrased from Hahnemann *Chronic Diseases,* Volume 1, pg. 125.

8. Hahnemann, *Chronic Diseases,* Volume 1, pg. 126.

CHAPTER 8

The Wisdom Of Waiting

All things oppose haste in prescribing.[1]

Apart from practicing patience, humility, and compassionate, unprejudiced observance, I think it's true to say, waiting is probably the most difficult and yet often, the most curative aspect of classical homoeopathy. Counter to common expectation, on many occasions waiting effectively reduces suffering and *hastens* cure. Frequently we often do just as good work waiting as when prescribing. Sometimes we may even do our very best work while waiting!

The material presented in the preceding Chapters 4 through 6 reveals the extent to which, during the second prescription phase, much of our success and failure depends on how well we understand and how skillfully we apply the rules of the homoeopathic waiting game.

I presume that most good prescribers will say: "We have often acted too soon, but never waited too long." Many physicians fail because of not waiting, and yet the waiting must be governed by knowledge . . . To know that this waiting is right is quite different from waiting without a fixed purpose.[2]

The concept of waiting will be harder for some than others. But often in homoeopathy there is much wisdom in waiting. Sure, we're waiting for something to happen, but we're also waiting *while* something is happening. Waiting in homoeopathy allows the vital force to work unhindered. Waiting prevents the practitioner from inadvertently interrupting the curative action of a medicine and avoids risking case confusion through untimely prescribing. Waiting actively allows us to watch the action of the vital force and avoid unnecessary patient suffering.

> The doctor watches the improvement of the patient and the corresponding disappearance of the symptoms under the first prescription, and when the case comes to a standstill he is uneasy, and with increasing fidgetiness he awaits the coming indication for the next dose of medicine. This fidgetiness which comes from a lack of knowledge unfits the physician as an observer and judge of symptoms; hence we see the doctor usually failing to cure his own children. He cannot wait and reason clearly over the returning symptoms.[3]

Since successful homoeopathy is always a patient-practitioner cooperative venture, watching and waiting is when we would do well to appeal to the patient's intellect. It works well to educate patients thoroughly in *their* healing process and enlist their informed agreement to watch and wait *together*. If necessary, we may offer appropriate, adjunctive support such as education, sympathy, and encouragement, and suggest undynamic analgesics such as soluble aspirin for severe pains or massage for aching joints. These supportive measures help reduce the impact of maintaining causes in the patient's life, but be careful not to overdo them and inadvertently confuse the picture. The very best help we can offer is accurate, careful, classical homoeopathic treatment.

Whenever in doubt about acting, never risk jeopardizing previous, intelligent work by not reasoning clearly. It pays dividends to take the time to meticulously examine the patient and the case.

> This flopping about, and not waiting for the remedy to cure is abominable. There are periods of improvement and failure. Let the Life Force go on as long as it can, and repeat only when the original [presenting] symptoms come back to stay.[4]

The more complex the case, the more especially important it is for the patient that we swallow pride, grasp humility by the neck, and ask a more experienced colleague for help. A different perspective often brings greater clarity to a complicated case.

Another golden key to effective homoeopathy is clarity of perception. Never prescribe until you perceive clearly and definitely the image of the remedy being called for by the state of the vital force, susceptibility, and predominant miasm.

Together, with perception, patience, and keen observation, personal integrity is of paramount importance in homoeopathy. Unless we are extremely disciplined and methodical we risk falling prey to the pressures of a busy practice and its time constraints. If we are under the gun, pressurized by the patient or driven by anxiety or impatience rather than our experience and reasoning, the ability to clearly perceive some small yet extremely significant shift in symptom pattern is in jeopardy. Consequently, we risk making the most frequently made mistake in homoeopathy *prescribing before the vital force is ready to proceed*, resulting in failure to cure because we confused the case. This is a sober thought for all of us, because in trying our best to help the patient we still make mistakes. The most important thing is to recognize the mistakes we have made and learn from them.

> Young practitioners and many old ones too, for that matter, give too many doses, repeat too frequently, change remedies too often. They give no time for reaction. They get doubtful, or hurried, or careless, and presently they get "rattled" if the case is serious. Then it is "all up with them" until or unless they come to their senses and correct their mistakes. Sometimes such mistakes cannot be corrected and a patient pays the penalty with his life.[5]

As we know, in all aspects of homoeopathic treatment, it's very important to comprehend that the patient's vital force is really in charge. We are in deep trouble if we don't realize that homoeopaths are in effect, servant scribes of the patient's vital force.

Decisions and actions after administration of the first prescription involve a skillful balancing act. We frequently walk a tightrope between waiting or prescribing the next remedy. Unfortunately, living in a high speed, modern society that virtually forbids illness and devastates us financially if we should dare fall ill, we are conditioned to go for the over-the-counter, quick fix, temporary relief. Quietly watching and waiting for the dynamic vital force to respond naturally and curatively at its own individual pace is a wholly different way to proceed and an extremely hard ball game for both patients and practitioners.

Let me give a simple recent example from my own practice: having successfully prescribed for a female patient, we met for our regular follow-up interview. Prior to this she had been improving rapidly on all levels. As I went to collect her from the waiting area, I observed that a huge wart-like growth had appeared on her face, the return of an old symptom. The patient was very anxious, because much of her work was in the public eye. Family, friends, and clients had urged her to do something about it immediately. We both felt pressurized to do something. I thought, if Hahnemann and Kent are right, because the remedy is acting as demonstrated by the continual rapid improvement in the case, I must wait.

It was all very well for me to think that, but what to say to the patient to encourage trust to this extent? And how long should I wait? According to Hahnemann's teachings, when the vital force is up and running we can trust it to carry on curing. I explained my understanding of the situation to the patient and together we decided to wait for two weeks and see what would happen. Two weeks later the patient returned. The growth had completely disappeared, without even scarring the skin. It is through cases like this we observe the power of homoeopathy in partnership with the vital force, and confirm how important it is to allow ourselves to be led by the teachings of Hahnemann and his close followers.

In essence the second prescription involves expertise, teamwork, and timing. After administration of the first prescription, the patient's health declines, improves, or doesn't change at all. Everything depends upon the practitioner's ability to perceive the true state of the individual, on the ability to correctly interpret the meaning of symptoms, which indicate the state of the vital force, level of resistance or susceptibility, and the active or dormant state of the inherited disease predispositions. Accurate interpretation of the information received leads to successful prescribing.

In the second prescription evaluation process, the practitioner weighs the need to prescribe against the need to watch and wait for the vital force to tell us what to do next. Effective practice of all the essential, professional skills—perception, observation, listening, and logical analysis, combined with a deep understanding of what we are doing and why, make the crucial difference between confusion or clarity, success or failure.

In maintaining the curative momentum, patient and practitioner become partners in an intricate and extraordinarily powerful dance, moving and responding to the rhythm of the vital force. Exhilarating, challenging, and endlessly rewarding, the second prescription phase of homoeopathic treatment is the true manifestation of the science, heart, and art of healing through Dr. Samuel Hahnemann's classical homoeopathy.

CHAPTER 8

1. Kent, *Minor Writings,* pg. 235.
2. Kent, *Minor Writings,* pg. 232.
3. Kent, *Minor Writings,* pg. 236.
4. Kent, *Lesser Writings,* pg. 675.
5. Close, *The Genius of Homoeopathy,* Chapter 13, pg. 203.

LITERATURE CITED

Allen, M.D., J. H. *The Chronic Miasms, Psora and Pseudo-Psora*. New Delhi, India: B. Jain Publishers Pvt. Ltd. Reprinted 1994.

Allen, M.D., T. F. *The Principles and Practicability of Boenninghausen's Therapeutic Pocket Book*. 5th American ed. New Delhi, India: B. Jain Publishers Pvt. Ltd.

Bidwell, M.D., Glen Irving. *How to Use the Repertory, with a Practical Analysis of Forty Homoeopathic Remedies*. New Delhi, India: Indian Books and Periodical Syndicate.

Boger, M.D., C. M. *Boenninghausen's Characteristics Materia Media & Repertory with Word Index*. 3rd ed. New Delhi, India: B. Jain Publishers Pvt. Ltd. Reprinted 1992.

Close M.D., Stuart. *The Genius of Homoeopathy. Lectures and Essays on Homoeopathic Philosophy*. New Delhi, India: B. Jain Publishers Pvt. Ltd. Reprinted 1991.

Dunham, Carroll, M.D. *Homoeopathy, The Science of Therapeutics*. New Delhi, India: Pratap Medical Publishers. First Indian ed.

Farrington, M.D., Harvey. *Homoeopathy and Homoeopathic Prescribing.* New Delhi, India: B. Jain Publishers Pvt. Ltd. Reprinted 1993.

Hahnemann, Dr. Samuel. *The Chronic Diseases, Their Peculiar Nature and Homoeopathic Cure.* 2nd ed. Pemberton Dudley, M.D., ed. New Delhi, India: B. Jain Publishers Pvt. Ltd. Reprinted 1994.

Hahnemann, Dr. Samuel. *Organon of Medicine.* 5th and 6th ed. Translated from the 5th ed. by R. E. Dudgeon, M.D., with additions and alterations as per sixth ed. translated by W. Boericke, M.D. New Delhi, India: B. Jain Publishers Pvt. Ltd. Reprinted 1992.

Hahnemann, Dr. Samuel. *Organon of Medicine. The Art of Healing.* 6th ed. Translated by W. Boericke, M.D. New Delhi, India: B. Jain Publishers Pvt. Ltd. Reprinted 1994.

Hahnemann, Dr. Samuel. *Organon of Medicine. The Art of Healing.* 5th ed. Translated by C. Wesselhoeft, M.D. New Delhi, India: B. Jain Publishers Pvt. Ltd. (Mistitled reprint of 6th American edition), 1988.

Hahnemann, Dr. Samuel. *Organon of Medicine.* Translated by J. Künzli, M.D., A. Naudé, and P. Pendleton. London, UK: Victor Gollancz Ltd. Published 1986.

Kent, A.M., M.D., James Tyler. *Kent's Final General Repertory of the Homoeopathic Materia Medica,* Eds. Pierre Schmidt, M.D., and Diwan Harish Chand, M.B., B.S. New Delhi, India: National Homoeopathic Pharmacy. Revised edition, 1980.

Kent, A.M., M.D., James Tyler, (date of first publication unknown). *New Remedies, Clinical Cases, Lesser Writings, Aphorisms, and Precepts.* W. W. Sherwood, ed. New Delhi, India: B. Jain Publishers Pvt. Ltd. Second reprint 1976.

Kent, A.M., M.D., James Tyler. *Lectures on Homoeopathic Philosophy.* North Atlantic Books, Berkeley, CA. Printed 1981.

Kent, A.M., M.D., James Tyler. *Kent's Minor Writings on Homoeopathy.* Compiled and edited by K. H. Gypser, M.D. Heidelberg, Germany: Karl F. Haug Publishers. Indian reprint, 1988, B. Jain Publishers Pvt. Ltd.

Roberts, M.D., Herbert A. *The Principles and Art of Cure by Homoeopathy. A Modern Textbook.* 2nd ed. New Delhi, India: B. Jain Publishers Ltd. Reprinted 1992.

Wright-Hubbard, M.D., Elizabeth. *A Brief Study Course in Homoeopathy.* St. Louis, MO: Formur, Inc. Fifth Printing 1992.

WEBSTER'S International Dictionary of the English Language, 1902, G. & C. Merriam & Co., Springfield, Mass. USA.

INDEX

A

acute 13, 24, 28, 34, 52, 53, 54, 55, 70, 71, 72, 73, 75, 86, 89, 99, 116, 117, 120, 145
affinities 100
aggravation 30, 31, 36, 48, 58, 59, 68, 72, 73, 74, 75, 87, 88, 89, 90, 91, 92, 113, 116, 122, 123, 124, 126, 127, 128, 139, 140
AIDS 6, 116
allopathic 116, 117, 138
alternating states 133, 134
alternation 6, 133, 134
amelioration 30, 48, 52, 58, 65, 67, 74, 84, 86, 87, 89, 104, 123, 125, 136, 138, 140
antidote 88, 92, 93, 97, 102, 105
artificial disease 123
attenuate 47, 100
attenuation 9, 98, 113

B

Boger 58

C

cancer 6, 116
case taking 5, 33, 40, 41, 73, 106
causation 5, 18, 36, 50, 51
central disturbance 28, 50, 80, 94
chronic 13, 24, 33, 34, 52, 54, 55, 68, 70, 71, 73, 75, 84, 85, 87, 89, 99, 114, 115, 116, 117, 120, 126, 131, 133, 145, 147

Chronic Diseases 2, 6, 46, 69, 97, 102, 134
Close 2, 40, 48, 51, 58, 91, 105, 134
complementary remedy 55, 99, 100, 133
curative 3, 8, 9, 10, 12, 19, 47, 48, 51, 117, 122, 125, 128,
    135, 136, 138, 140, 141, 144, 145, 149, 150, 153, 154

D

decline 23, 24, 29, 35, 39, 67, 86, 88, 89, 154
defense mechanism 5, 30
degree of progress 35
diluted 91, 122
dilution 9, 119, 120, 122, 127
Direction of Cure 12, 13, 14, 25, 30, 40, 50, 51, 55, 59, 74, 76,
    77, 92, 96, 103, 138
disease 2, 3, 5, 6, 7, 8, 9, 10, 12, 15, 16, 17, 19, 20, 24, 31, 32,
    46, 47, 49, 50, 51, 52, 54, 58, 59, 66, 69, 70, 71, 72, 73,
    75, 78, 82, 83, 87, 89, 90, 91, 92, 93, 96, 97, 101, 102,
    104, 105, 114, 115, 121, 123, 124, 126, 127, 128, 131,
    134, 138, 139, 147, 154
dosage 9, 10, 27, 30, 39, 45, 47, 58, 86, 113, 116, 120, 121
doses 8, 11, 66, 70, 71, 91, 107, 113, 114, 116, 117, 120, 121,
    122, 125, 128, 135, 141, 152
Dunham 2
dynamization 7, 9, 113, 114, 115, 119, 120
dynamized 7, 47, 100

E

energy 2, 37, 38, 76, 96, 98
excitation 59, 69, 72, 78, 88, 124
exteriorization 32, 54, 59
exteriorize 30, 32, 59, 73, 83, 89, 138

F

Farrington 58
first prescription 1, 10, 23, 24, 25, 26, 28, 32, 41, 46, 57, 61,
    63, 65, 66, 76, 79, 85, 92, 93, 94, 95, 106, 131, 134, 135,
    136, 150, 152, 154

O

observations 26, 27, 28, 48, 114
organism 2, 4, 5, 6, 7, 17, 25, 30, 33, 38, 46, 47, 48, 54, 67,
    68, 82, 83
Organon 2, 3, 7, 8, 11, 15, 16, 19, 21, 29, 46, 82, 104, 113,
    115, 119, 127, 134
original case 35, 37, 40, 136

P

palliative 28, 32, 51, 57
partial 15, 96, 101, 106, 140
partial prescription 85
partials 104
pathognomonic 32, 48
pathology 5, 42, 53, 83, 89, 90, 91, 93, 140
pattern of change 35
peculiar symptoms 71, 104
perceive 4, 9, 12, 16, 19, 28, 40, 90, 138, 140, 151, 152, 154
perceived 5, 35, 47, 84, 117, 122
placebo 24, 146
potency 1, 9, 11, 12, 26, 27, 31, 33, 45, 47, 53, 55, 59, 60, 63,
    67, 71, 75, 76, 77, 79, 85, 86, 87, 88, 89, 90, 93, 95, 96,
    97, 98, 113, 114, 115, 116, 117, 118, 121, 122, 128, 132,
    136, 138, 139, 140, 144
principles 1, 2, 13, 14, 18, 19, 40, 91, 94, 106
prognosis 13, 23, 54, 140
progress chart 41, 42
progress report 33, 68, 76
provings 8, 9, 47, 82, 139
psoric 6, 69, 70, 89, 97, 102, 133, 134, 141

R

relapse 140
related remedies 133
repertory 81, 99, 106, 145
return of old symptoms 24, 30, 78, 95, 101, 103, 132
return of presenting symptoms 65, 123

S

second prescription 1, 2, 3, 9, 10, 12, 14, 18, 23, 25, 26, 27,
    28, 41, 45, 55, 60, 68, 80, 93, 131, 133, 145, 146, 149,
    154
single dose 26, 63, 100, 143
succession of remedies 99
succussion 9, 119, 120, 121, 123, 128
suppressive 28, 32, 51, 99, 138
susceptibility 3, 4, 5, 6, 7, 8, 12, 30, 53, 57, 58, 63, 65, 77,
    121, 138, 139, 151, 154
symptom shift 36
symptom timeline 50

T

totality 7, 8, 11, 14, 15, 16, 17, 18, 24, 32, 39, 47, 53, 59, 81,
    85, 87, 94, 95, 96, 99, 105, 117, 137, 138, 140
tubercular 6, 51

U

unprejudiced observer 28, 29

V

vital force 2, 3, 5, 6, 8, 9, 10, 12, 13, 16, 23, 24, 25, 27, 30, 32,
    35, 38, 46, 47, 49, 53, 55, 59, 60, 63, 64, 66, 67, 68, 71,
    73, 76, 77, 80, 82, 83, 87, 88, 89, 90, 97, 98, 99, 100, 101,
    115, 117, 120, 121, 125, 126, 134, 136, 138, 139, 140,
    143, 144, 145, 150, 151, 152, 153, 154
vitality 37, 67, 87, 88, 116, 140

W

wait 60, 62, 65, 66, 67, 69, 73, 74, 75, 77, 79, 93, 102, 103,
    135, 139, 141, 143, 144, 145
waiting 23, 24, 49, 53, 57, 64, 65, 76, 102, 105, 132, 141,
    144, 146, 149, 150, 151, 152, 153

TOTALITY PRESS
INSTITUTE OF CLASSICAL HOMOEOPATHY

TOTALITY PRESS IS THE PUBLISHING branch of the Institute of Classical Homoeopathy, a non-profit educational institution dedicated to furthering the highest standards of homoeopathic medicine, through publishing, research, and education.

Totality Press publishes books for homoeopathic practitioners, students, and the general public.

The Institute of Classical Homoeopathy offers a comprehensive academic and clinical homoeopathic training, introductory lectures and specialized courses, and operates a free homoeopathic clinic in San Francisco.

For more information about Totality Press or the Institute of Classical Homoeopathy, contact:

Phone: (415) 248-1632
Fax: (707) 963-6131
Visit our website at: www.classicalhomoeopathy.org

Or write us at:
1336-D Oak Avenue
St. Helena, CA 94574
U.S.A.

2nd Prescription

Vital to assess accurately the
outcome of first prescription on
the symptoms first described by px
Lose sight of the signs of vital force
& we cant help px.

In (h) cure takes place because we
are as similarly susceptible to the
homeopathic medicine chosen as
we are to the stimulus that disturbed
us (trauma, environment, change in
temp, diet, how we react to offense,
loss, love, joy etc.

The way we measure susceptibility
is assessing how px responds, reacts
& adapts to various internal & external
stimuli — or a px survival technique,
in other words.
Susceptibility describes the state of
the vital force at any given moment
in time. If the vital force was described
as a face, susceptability will be the
expression on the face. So
susceptability is the observed
change in the VF through symptoms since
ill health occurred. The Px unique coping
response to stimulis in the context of his
life circumstances & sx patterns.

...re indicated thru the pax expressio
... & family health history.
appropriate
a remedy suitable to px miasm
prescribing.

...at which has the power to harm, has
the power to heal' (Law of similars)
Hippocrates.

Remedies shud match as an 'artificial'
disease the sxs of the px's original
disease. Dynamization of (H) medicines
renders them energetically stronger than
the original degree and can therefore
cancell the original disease and to
act directly on susceptibility of vital force.
They target & resemble the state of the
vital force, correspond to the
predominant miasm & satisfy pxs
susceptability, thus helping VF to
restore its equilibrium.

* In 2nd presc. read again data in mat med
related to action of 1st prescription & how
they relate to curative potential of
selected remedy.